# PRIVATE PHYSIOTHERAPY

MY JOURNEY AND YOUR JOURNEY
TOWARDS SUCCESSFULLY PRACTISING
PHYSIOTHERAPY PRIVATELY

## Gal Kantor

*BSc Physiotherapy, MSc Manual Therapy*
*HCPC, MCSP, MMACP*

U K Book Publishing.com

Editing, design, typesetting and publishing by UK Book Publishing

www.ukbookpublishing.com

ISBN: 978-1-914195-50-1

# PRIVATE PHYSIOTHERAPY

# CONTENTS

**PREFACE**     **1**

**INTRODUCTION**     **5**

Who This Book Is for     5

Starting Your Journey     5

**1 – MY JOURNEY**     **9**

Private Practice: A Pathway to Success     10

My One-Man Practice Solution     12

**2 – BECOMING A PRIVATE PHYSIOTHERAPIST**     **15**

A Huge Professional Decision     15

Becoming a Genuinely Proficient Physiotherapist     18

Moving into the Private Sector     20

Keep On Moving to Keep On Growing     22

**3 – QUALIFICATIONS, QUALIFICATIONS, QUALIFICATIONS**     **26**

MSKP and MT     26

**4 – ESTABLISHMENT, MANAGEMENT AND MONEY MATTERS**     **32**

Your Skill Set and Your Business's Image     35

Private Practice Attitudes     36

Building a Practice with Little or No Money     39

Moving to a Real Practice     42

Employing Trainees, Junior Physiotherapists or Senior

  Physiotherapists     47

    Rule 1     49

    Rule 2     49

    Rule 3     49

    Rule 4     50

Rule 5                                                              50
Rule 6                                                              50
Managing and Balancing Your Private Practice Finances              52
Work, Lifestyle and Life Balance                                  56

## 5 – PROFESSIONAL AND PERSONAL SKILLS                            62

Working Alone Effectively                                          62
Social Skills inside the Practice                                  64
How to Work Fast in a Crowded Schedule                            66
Safe yet Effective Practice                                        70
Communicative Skills                                               74
Solving Physical Problems                                         77
Fast Clinical Reasoning                                           78
Delivering Real Value during Treatments                          80

## 6 – IMPROVING EVERY PATIENT IMMEDIATELY                         82

Integrating Clinical Approaches into Your Practice                82
The Maitland® Approach                                            85
Cyriax's Orthopaedic Medicine                                     86
Applied Kinesiology                                               87
Using Exercises Accurately and Effectively                        89
Treating with Technology Devices                                  91
Finding and Using Cutting-Edge Technology                         93
Intensified Professional Development                              97

## 7 – MARKETING YOUR BEST SELF                                   102

Your Competition—Who Else Is Out There                           102
The Chiropractor                                             103
The Osteopath                                                104
The Sports Therapist                                         105
The Masseur                                                  106
The Alternative Therapist                                    106
Dealing with Your Competitors                                    108
Word of Mouth                                                    110

Building your Own Client Database                                114

Marketing Tools                                                  118

    One                                      120

    Two                                      120

    Three                                    120

Websites and More about Online Marketing                         124

The Slow Periods                                                 129

Value-Based Prices                                               131

Becoming the Very Best Practitioner–for Your Client              136

Protecting Your Reputation                                       138

Should You Expand?                                               142

## 8 – CLIENTS: YOUR GREATEST ASSET                              146

Valued Private Clients                                           146

Dealing with Assumed High-Profile Clients                        148

Clients with Complex Conditions                                  150

Dealing with Difficult Clients                                   154

Avoiding Complaints and Dealing with Them                        156

Looking After Your Clients                                       162

Attracting and Inspiring Clients                                 163

## 9 – AFTERWORDS                                                165

Your Future                                                      165

The Future of Private Physiotherapy                              167

The Post COVID-19 Private Practice                               171

# PREFACE

F irst and foremost, thank you for deciding to read my book. I feel fulfilled when a physiotherapist–or any healthcare practitioner–takes the time to look inside it. I truly believe that what you'll read and learn from me here is important and helpful for all of us who practise our profession, in the public and private sectors alike. It has been suggested to me that the term 'private' to describe physiotherapy work should be replaced by 'independent'–for sector, physiotherapy or physiotherapist. Hence, my choice to use the term 'private' is completely personal. The use of this term in this book is not intended to disrespect or undermine the public sector and its much-needed services. My work and services ('privately' or 'independently') have always gone hand in hand with the public services and their dedicated professionals.

My clear view and professional experience as a private practice owner and practitioner, along with my genuine aim to deliver them here through this book, will hopefully increase the success rate of treatment delivered by physiotherapists in the private and the public sectors alike. Helping to make physiotherapists better in a few key aspects and thereby improving their regular rate of successful treatment outcomes would undoubtedly mean happier and healthier clients. It also means taking some pressure off the often-overloaded public services by preventing or reducing the need for certain surgeries and more minor medical procedures and by helping to avoid long-term chronic and complex conditions, all of which public healthcare services often end up dealing with. This book refers to and discusses the private work which I am specialised in, but the core elements of practising the physiotherapy profession as I describe it here can be applied to us all, everywhere and at any career stage.

The thoughts I share with you in this book are based on what I've done so far and what worked for me. They therefore aim to help you as a fellow physiotherapist at any stage of your career, whether you're already a private practitioner, are aiming towards becoming one, or even if you're still practising in the public sector. I'm confident the tips and guidance I provide you with will turn your journey to private practice from a vague aspiration into a concrete plan.

My name is Gal Kantor. I'm a physiotherapist who deals mainly with clients who suffer from musculoskeletal (MSK) conditions, specialising in manual therapy and the management of sports injuries. Every day, just as you do, I treat patients. I truly enjoy and love my work, but apart from that, what qualifies me to write this book?

First, I hold several qualifications in the physiotherapy profession and sport, with particular interest and experience in swimming. Second, I guest-lecture at Glasgow Caledonian University, in the Department of Health and Social Care, and I occasionally supervise physiotherapy students, as well as deliver different forms of professional affiliation here in Glasgow. Third, I run my own educational courses and workshops online and offline at my clinic, all of which I have developed and refined over the years.

Fourth, my professional experience includes public health services, yet it is mostly within the private sector and at sports events–regionally, nationally, and up to international and Olympic levels.

Incidentally though, what I write about is not based solely on my personal experience. To make this book even more comprehensive and reliable, I've discussed the issues involved with many professionals in my field. Finally, I have studied the profession full-time as an undergraduate–and part-time as a postgraduate. I then started my businesses, then owned and managed my own successful practice, GK Physiotherapy. I've intermittently hired a qualified physiotherapist and taught and trained alongside myself students and qualified trainees. Yet for most of my career, I've worked joyfully by myself as a one-man dedicated brand, all in all for approximately 20 years by the time of

This book is not a promising roadmap for setting up a multi-million automated business system. Its aim is to mentor you in developing and adopting your private practice ethos. That includes giving you guidance about what I believe is:

- the most relevant professional development;
- how to set up your practice so you hit the ground running; and
- crucial tips about delivering and marketing your (unique) services.

I conclude with an extensive section about the many types of patients I've treated and how I've interacted with them in a mutually beneficial way.

> My ethos is to provide superior services in a pleasant and professional atmosphere to all my clients. In this book I show you how I've done this.

I also discuss the virtues of practising efficiently in an enjoyable and rewarding physiotherapy environment, which is often not the reality for many practitioners who work publicly or even privately, under the pressure of an extreme caseload and endless waiting lists.

In short, this book is about how I became successful in delivering world-class private physiotherapy in an ethical, balanced and rewarding manner. How you use this book is up to you, but I'm certain it will provide you with the essential outlook, knowledge and a good number of tools to achieve the same–and hopefully far more!

At this point, I wish to convey my heartfelt gratitude to everyone who has helped me throughout my long educational and professional career and in the long process of completing this book: my university tutors, course leaders and supervisors, fellow students, professional tutors and practice owners who taught and trained me, my trainees, editing specialists who have helped me complete and publish this book, and of course some good friends, and to my family, who have supported me throughout.

*Yours professionally and truthfully,*
**Gal.**

# INTRODUCTION

———————●———————

## Who This Book Is for

I f you're already a private practitioner, this book will help you understand where you are right now. If you're a physiotherapist working for someone else or within the public health services, doing the same job every day and earning the same amount regardless of your knowledge, skills, efficiency and hard work, this book will move you on to your next level.

## Starting Your Journey

Before I point you to the issues and problems that motivated me to write this book on private physiotherapy, I'd like to ask you a few key questions:

- Are you happy with where you work?
- Do you enjoy your daily physiotherapy job?
- Is your current job secure?
- Are you happy with what you earn?
- Would you like to double–or triple–your income?
- Have you ever dreamed of working for yourself?
- Would you like to significantly increase your income?
- Would you like more flexible control over your lifestyle?
- Is owning your own private practice part of your professional or personal aspiration?

If you're looking to work for yourself in a profession you love, then I can help you realise your dream. I can help you by telling you about my personal and professional experience in private physiotherapy, public health, and the educational sector—about how I realised my dream.

Once upon a time I asked myself those same questions. I discovered that I believed in myself and my abilities: I could achieve my professional dreams. My day-to-day life is a living proof.

I'm not saying getting to where I am today was easy, or that I accomplished it all without a struggle. But I always felt it was worthwhile to pursue my professional goals in tandem with my personal goals, so my overall achievements are more complete and more rounded.

*** 

People have different motivations in their professional careers—some may dream of retiring and travelling the world; others may be more focused on building a scaleable and saleable business.

I wonder what your motivation is?

But whatever it is, I promise you that by maintaining reasonable financial discipline—along with some common and conscious investment actions—you should achieve a degree of financial independence well before you reach retirement age. Just imagine.

In this book I'll talk you through the aspects of what I have accomplished which can help you achieve your goals. The model I'm going to share with you is appealing, realistic and rewarding—regardless of the stage you are currently at in your professional life.

---

**If you want to achieve your own level of success as a private practitioner, I am confident I can help you.**

---

You can start by learning from how I did it, then perhaps later on you can draw on your own strengths to succeed in ways that lie beyond your wildest imagination at the moment.

In this new professional environment of private physiotherapy I'll introduce you to, you'll acquire every professional element and related interactive communicative tools required to deliver what I regard as outstanding physiotherapy services. You can deliver this expertise to your clients at the best price and at a level they will immediately value. Their satisfaction levels will be so high they will automatically recommend you to their friends, family and colleagues.

Eventually, you will also earn a different level of comfortable income for as long as you wish to practise in your field. You'll be able to take time off and go on long holidays–and your clients will be waiting for you when you return. Your phone will keep ringing with calls from returning clients months or even years after you've stopped practising–if you ever choose to do so. Therefore, you'll be much less likely to lose your job, your clients and your core practice.

Please throw away any preconceptions about whether a 'hands-off' approach works better than a 'hands-on' approach. Forget what you were told about manipulations being too risky or that exercises don't work. Forget about fixed salaries or the myth that only by becoming a ward manager or pursuing a certain professional grade or hire a full team to work for you can you achieve high earnings. Forget about working nine-to-five, too. You may work longer hours, but that will be your choice; you will be well rewarded for it and will enjoy working harder and longer when you want or need to.

The information in this book can tell you everything you need to know about every area of my own private practice work. Yet, even if you don't plan to work for yourself or to open your own practice over the short term, why not take the first step and read this book through? Read it all and start planning your own route towards working as a private physiotherapist in the independent healthcare sector.

# Finally, remember very few physiotherapists ever fulfil their dream of practising both privately and successfully, which I now truly hope you will!

Therefore, if you feel inspired by what you have read so far, you might decide to become one of the lucky few to build a successful private practice.

# 1 – MY JOURNEY

M y story is no fairy tale. It was far from easy to get to where I am today. I was a busy competitive swimmer back in my youth, and so my school grades were average and just too low to qualify to study physiotherapy back in my own country– and I had no money (and I mean absolutely none) to even consider studying abroad. I had to go to work to earn a living and save money. At age 23 I was a hard-driven, hard-working young man, armed with a lot of life experience, but with nothing to fulfil my dream of becoming a physiotherapist, never mind a chance of doing it in a foreign country, in a foreign language.

After failing in my second attempt to achieve the entry requirements and grades required to study physiotherapy in my home country, I decided to move on and approach it in my own way.

I educated myself as a lifeguard and swimming coach, and in the process learned a lot about swimming pool maintenance. During the summers of 1999 and 2000 I worked around pools, doing maintenance jobs, teaching and coaching swimming, both to beginners and to competitive swimmers. In between times I travelled, taking whatever jobs came my way and all the time learning and improving my use of English.

I got into a school of physiotherapy in the very east of Holland, but before the end of my second year I ran out of money. I reluctantly accepted my parents' support for a few months, but my pride wouldn't let me consider this as anything but a short-term fix.

I was close to being a stony-broke, starving student when a good Dutch friend found me a job: outdoor physical labour in the rough Dutch weather on a huge plantation. Although I had begun studying Dutch from the time I arrived, I still understood very little of it by then but was grateful for the additional income. I'll never forget finishing my first day of work knowing I could actually afford to buy food at the supermarket. I could now keep body and soul together, and I managed to track down additional student grants that I used to successfully complete my studies. After four years' study in Holland, I became a fully qualified physiotherapist, and I was also trained to work in the Dutch language.

There were other struggles and useful lessons I learned from them between then and now: professional accreditations earned in other countries, professional exams as part of completing my master's degree, and numerous professional memberships. I lectured and taught in a university for the first time at the same time as making tough yet rewarding business and professional decisions. I'll summarise these as I go along so you can learn from my experience.

# Private Practice: A Pathway to Success

From my very first year of physiotherapy studies in Holland, I knew I wanted to treat people in a private practice setting. Some of my teachers at the university were what used to be called 'manual therapists', which means they were officially trained and specialised in MSK conditions within physiotherapy.

They consistently demonstrated a superb level of clinical reasoning and manual skills, way beyond the average capabilities of other physiotherapists who practised privately or publicly around them. Their successful image within the profession and their skills attracted my attention from the outset. These skilled manual therapists could also handle sports injuries very well, but mostly they were also private practitioners who ran their own practices around the city.

I'll never forget a Swiss friend of mine, an excellent student named Heidi, who was studying physiotherapy in the year above me. She had just come home after a clinical placement with a manual therapist–and she told me this: 'Gal, manual therapy works!'

It was then I decided on my ultimate goal: to become a manual therapist myself and to someday open my own private practice.

I wanted to associate myself with every well-educated and experienced practitioner who would agree to take me on, even for just a day. In order to learn new skills and gather knowledge, I was ready to do absolutely anything for them for free. Watching them work made me appreciate what it takes to be a truly successful private practitioner in the eyes of clients and colleagues.

> **I realised it was extremely important to develop strong clinical reasoning skills, as well as strong manual skills. However, it took much more than that to achieve the level of success I had in mind, which I will explain later on.**

I went on observing and learning from the best physiotherapy professionals I knew, both during and after my studies. It is hard to express my respect for–and my gratitude to–these people who so generously gave of their time and freely shared with me their valuable, hard-earned experience.

After all these years of observing and learning from so many different professionals, I sometimes compare physiotherapy to cooking: you can learn wonderful recipes from almost anyone– regardless of credentials, professional experience or skill level. I always find learning a new physiotherapy 'recipe' incredibly exciting.

It took five years of part-time postgraduate studies to achieve my master's degree in Manual Therapy and to gain prestigious membership of the Manipulative/Musculoskeletal Association of Chartered Physiotherapists (MACP; the term 'Manipulative' has recently changed to 'Musculoskeletal.) Of course, learning never stops. Besides numerous short-term continuing education courses, I also spent the next ten years completing over ten course modules offered by Moscow University's Department of Manual Therapy in order to gain full professional confidence in this field.

# My One-Man Practice Solution

The good news I have for you is that you don't necessarily need to spend years and years learning at postgraduate level. You don't need to study for academic degrees and pay for lots of expensive courses the way I did.

If you wish to perform brilliantly in the eyes of your clients, then you need to be very careful about picking the knowledge and skills you 'take in' on the one hand and what you actually 'deliver out' to your customers on the other.

You will discover that your professional development can be specific and targeted to private clients. That can save you years of studying unnecessary skills. Instead, you can focus your efforts on what works well for you and on the knowledge that lets you achieve the best results in private practice as well as the public sector.

We can't spend our entire time studying, taking every course and going to every seminar.

> **Our money and time resources are limited and so we all need to plan our professional development down to the smallest detail.**

You will love your learning pathway I will tell you about – but the private practice concept, as a whole, will need to be clarified as being different in the way it is practised with patients and the way it is managed.

I explain and discuss this subject in more detail in the next chapter.

I've written this book to show you exactly how I achieved my private practice dreams and to make sure you understand how you can also achieve them too, while thoroughly *enjoying* the journey.

Let's be clear: the aim of this book is not to lecture you on how to grow your business larger than your own capacity to be it and in it yourself and managing it yourself – though a few sections discuss this aspect pragmatically. I can't make you a multimillionaire business owner either, but I know for a fact that you will enjoy business success if you take the recommended steps I set out.

At one point I tried very hard to build up a true money-making business, but this attempt was expensive and gave me nothing but headaches; in the end I was left financially broke *and* unhappy.

If you want to make lots of money, running a large business is not a bad idea. However, if you wish to stay inside the profession, then you'd do well to learn from my mistakes and make different choices, at least while you start your private physiotherapy career. My suggestions are likely to make you much better off and more financially secure than almost any other physiotherapist around you–and sooner rather than later. However, we're not here to look at other people's success, wealth or happiness: only yours. This is about you, and what you want.

I firmly believe that earning large sums of money comes as a by-product of constant development in a certain direction, in combination with the right attitude, firm decisions and a set of realistic actions you can take as you go along. Later on, I will reveal tools and methods that will enable you to increase your actual and potential income significantly.

I urge you not to put off pursuing your dream.

---

## As you read this book, start taking steps to become a successful private practitioner.

---

At the same time as continuing your daily job and routine you can also start planning a pathway to help some individuals who need you to move towards a pain-free life–and also generate the income you deserve, love your job, work with great clients, handle interesting cases, and do all this according to your own flexible schedule.

You don't need to own your practice or to work in private practice to start using the information in this book. You can start at your local health centre or hospital, with your colleagues or friends.

While you read this book, you can take immediate action by treating friends, colleagues and family members, which will help you get your initial database organised. Start treating your daily clients as if they were private clients who are paying you directly; imagine how much they would pay for your treatment, think about asking them if you served them well enough to take their money. Try this out–but there is so much more to come.

## Start thinking private and develop an independent attitude now.

Act and behave as if you already own and run your own practice at your workplace, or wherever you are or operate from. Aim to demonstrate a higher sense of responsibility and level of care to your patients and to your work in general. Start presenting yourself well personally and professionally–in short, start building your own reputation.

Read on to build your 'private practice physiotherapy' skills and get yourself ready to gain knowledge and develop a professional career as a private physiotherapist.

I hope you'll enjoy your journey towards career autonomy in the private healthcare sector of physiotherapy!

# 2 – BECOMING A PRIVATE PHYSIOTHERAPIST

●

## A Huge Professional Decision

The biggest career decision you as a physiotherapist need to take is choosing the area of physiotherapy that you want to work and specialise in. This choice determines which direction is right for you.

## Decide early on which area you want to specialise in.

Modern physiotherapy education presents the entire profession to students over the course of three or four years. The specific technical content, approach and focus vary, of course, depending on the institution, the country and the programme. But in the end, it always requires the student to develop new levels of knowledge, communication and practical skills.

In contrast, very few of the practical skills you require to develop and run a private practice—such as business management for self-employment—feature in an undergraduate core curriculum.

Yet, many graduates decide on their professional focus and precise field of practice right after graduation—and they often base this crucial decision on their first professional job, whether or not they find it interesting or compatible with their personality and goals.

The more time passes, the harder it becomes for a new professional to change a path mapped out at the beginning. The result is that, instead of trying to satisfy a personal need they start searching for another job doing much the same but one they might like better ... that might pay a higher salary ... that might include a step onto the management ladder. And so they keep the treadmill in motion.

Often, when working for the first few years in the public sector, a graduate rotates through the different fields of physiotherapy in order to acquire professional experience. However, this rotation does little to nurture a person who is hoping to open a private practice, which requires a certain set of skills and a particular attitude you won't find in the public sector.

On the other hand, this is not to say that postgraduate work experience in different physiotherapy areas is not required. Far from it. Every physiotherapist needs to develop some kind of postgraduate experience, whether during job rotations within various physiotherapy disciplines in the public health service at home, or by travelling and gaining it abroad.

When I see a fresh graduate open a new full-time practice, I sometimes feel concerned for them –and for their clients–regardless of how successful they may have been in their studies or how prepared for it they felt at the point of graduation. Once your private practice is open, it can increase the pressure on you and leave little time for professional development–or self-development–in other areas.

Every graduate may need a wider range of initial professional experience as a physiotherapist. Setting up a business and trying to make money right away doesn't allow you to develop either your core clinical experience or those enhanced skills that privately paying clients often expect, appreciate and are ready to pay for. Developing the right level of skills takes commitment, dedication and the right attitude. And it takes time, which new business owners often spend worrying about receipts and invoices or constantly marketing their services.

# From my experience, it is crucial to choose a particular physiotherapy area very early on.

My own career decision, taken at the start of my career, was to specialise in the management of clients with Musculoskeletal (MSK) conditions through a Manual Therapy (MT) approach. As briefly mentioned earlier, MT used to be MSK's more traditional professional term, when practitioners would undergo advanced training to apply manipulative therapies based on advanced clinical reasoning and diagnostic thought processes. MT, therefore, originally referred to postgraduate development of the more basic MSK physiotherapy (MSKP), which is trained and used across the profession. Henceforth I'll use its more complete and comprehensive version, MSKP/MT. Just as I did, you need to build up your experience by observing people working, treating and handling caseloads, running practices and departments, and getting yourself ready to grow your career based on genuine professional judgement and hands-on experience.

To work in the private sector, and to do it efficiently, you need to master some key skills–and gaining these skills and developing your knowledge requires a massive investment of time and effort.

And beyond time and effort, it may also be expensive, especially if you choose certain postgraduate educational pathways–and in particular if you discover that your first choice is not right for you. However, making a firm decision about the exact area in which you wish to specialise is vital to becoming as prepared as possible to open a private practice.

While you can pick up valuable work experience in different disciplines–neurology, orthopaedics, paediatric physiotherapy, among others–you must always have your pathway to private physiotherapy firmly mapped out in your mind: specific learning activities and actions must support this goal.

By making an early decision to specialise in MSKP/MT, I started out to gain expertise in areas that would eventually allow me to deliver the best exercise therapies, manipulative treatments and sports-injury practice to my clients. You should do the same to work towards your own specialisation.

Do not wait until you have gained enough overall experience to make this major decision that MSKP/MT is your desired field of expertise. You can continue to pick up relevant experience as you make the early progress necessary to your career. Life is far too short to delay your ambitions and goals.

# Becoming a Genuinely Proficient Physiotherapist

I strongly recommend that you acquire multidisciplinary physiotherapy experience *before* treating people privately on a regular basis or opening a place of your own. Then consider taking the leap towards a private practice only once you have observed and learned from reputable private practitioners.

Your goal as a private practitioner is to become proficient in what you do with your clients. You also want them to think you're the best practitioner around, even though you may still have some way to go to learn and develop all the skills you need.

You can certainly start out working in private practice as an associate or employee–or even run some part-time services in the private sector. In my opinion, however, it is a mistake to have your business up and running too early, just for the sake of making money and owning a practice. While you can still work on your own, at an early stage–long before your skill levels fully mature–if you do it in the right way, your experience and learning curve will increase dramatically.

There are many ways to start very early and work by yourself, and still become an excellent physiotherapist. I'll explain this in later chapters. However, when it came to the more common aspiration of developing a larger business and handling different management rules and tasks, I was facing challenges which held back my actual development as a proficient physiotherapist.

During my career as a private practitioner, I have employed and mentored junior physiotherapists for short to medium terms, part- and full-time. They had little or no experience in private practice–and sometimes no experience at all. Some of them were exceptionally good with clients, and they developed their skills and gathered experience during the time they spent with me in my practice.

I've tutored, worked with and employed a wide variety of students and professionals, all of them with different abilities. In the long run, though, trying to expand beyond being a single professional in a one-person practice didn't work well for me–for a number of different reasons.

One involved a necessary trade-off: I had to give up the clinical side of the practice in exchange for training and managing other people who lacked clinical and practical experience to one degree or another, whether they were qualified, trainees or associates. Some of them were good enough to pull their own weight in the practice, though soon enough they were on their way to build their own careers in other directions. Hence the people I've employed and trained developed professionally, whereas I as the business owner or employer developed in a somewhat different pathway or into different areas of more interpersonal and managerial skills.

## Most clinicians only develop the ability to react quickly and efficiently during treatment over time.

It takes time to learn how to approach a client, immediately connect with them and then deliver skills efficiently. This can all be learned and developed–but it can't be taught, from scratch, on the frontline of a private practice. Lack of experience sticks out like a sore thumb and it often puts paying clients right off, whether they are regulars or people seeking help in your clinic for the first time.

I believe that graduates who set up private businesses early on in their careers can find themselves limited to the new business they started up and associated with. Therefore, I highly recommend taking on part-time work, shadowing, or finding a learning-experience programme. This can be a tremendous help to you as a practitioner at the start of your career.

Professional attitude and skills development have enormous value in the eyes of clients and can lead to word-of-mouth recommendations. Hence, becoming so proficient that clients talk about you requires social and practical skills that not many of your peers will be able to match.

We'll explore these particular skills and how to get them in ensuing chapters, but I suggest you remember right from the start, and always thereafter, that you must be good at what you do: you must be good with people; you need the ability to deliver what you promise in order to sell your skills to your customers.

Make no mistake. You should look after your clients. I will explain how and exactly who they are later on. But be aware that they will not give you a second thought if you have a poor skill set. They don't have time for amateurs or 'wannabe' private physiotherapists. You have to be truly proficient to excel here–and I will show you, throughout this book, how you can do exactly that.

# Moving into the Private Sector

Starting to work privately is not something you do just because you feel like it, or when you suddenly become dissatisfied with your profession, your job or your current colleagues. It is an important and a life-changing decision; it requires a commitment to an ongoing process of development that will lead you towards your next, or even your final, professional and financial goals as a private practitioner.

Ideally, you should start working towards your professional goals while studying for your basic physiotherapy degree by affiliating yourself in various places, or even working in private practices on a part-time basis. I used to observe and assist private practitioners, and each one was an experienced and respected manual therapist.

Some of my chosen university assignments or modules, including my final dissertations, related to MSKP/MT and the clinical reasoning that supports it. And so, very early on, I developed an understanding of how private practices worked and what it took to succeed as a private physiotherapist. I didn't need to wait until my first job to learn the basics; I was able to be helpful and productive in the practices I joined right at the beginning of my career.

Therefore, if you work towards your professional goals as I did, by the time you graduate you will already have some skills under your belt that will equip you to deliver effective treatments safely, make sure clients are comfortable, AND be assured that they appreciate your services. And you should be able to provide valuable skills and real help to any private practitioner you approach, or wish to be affiliated with, while you gain your personal experience.

As a trainee student who enrolled on an accredited pathway, it is important not to pressure your physiotherapist mentor, clinical instructor or the practice manager at your affiliation site to pay you wages, even if you think you deserve a certain amount of compensation for your work. Remember, you're there to learn–and you shouldn't expect a professional to pay *you* for being your teacher. You are exchanging some supervised work to gain experience and knowledge; understanding the value of this deal may well lead in the future to a job offer in that very clinic.

On the other hand, if you've asked to stay longer (or over a summer holiday period) or have gained the status of a novice or intern who brings sufficient skills and experience to fulfil a key role in the practice and are helping the owner to generate revenue, it is appropriate to discuss being reimbursed for travel and living expenses, in light of your value to the clinic.

Bear in mind that the effort you put in will be worth it only if the experience is of clear professional or personal value to you.

Having been a clinical affiliation host myself, I strongly advise you to ask your potential host for a very limited number of work experience hours in total to start with. Once you two have met and get on, then requesting a full-term curriculum placement would be more than appropriate. A trainee in a practice can be both demanding and tiring for the tutor, so it's important to limit your affiliation to agreed-upon times, being sure not to overstay your welcome. There's a world of difference between being a help and a hindrance to your host, having your tutor happy to help out or resentful of your presence. Unless agreed in advance, a simple request for a drop more of your tutor's time or asking to extend your affiliation period longer and beyond the previous agreement can swing the balance against you.

## Keep On Moving to Keep On Growing

Though you might imagine I would recommend you to apply for a full-time job in a small private practice as your very first job, I actually believe you'd be better served by taking the time to move around different workplaces, to learn as much as you can from different physiotherapists, whether in private practice or the state health services.

It goes without saying–though I will say it anyway–that you should always express your gratitude at the end of a learning opportunity. This holds true when you finish working for someone, whether or not you were offered employment, and regardless of how pleasant–or unpleasant–you found the work.

The experience you gain may well prove invaluable and may garner you job satisfaction and high income in the future. I am indebted for a great part of my career to some very senior professionals who agreed to teach me by letting me inside their core businesses. They allowed me to watch and understand how they run their practices, and to observe and often even to treat their own patients. Overall, they willingly shared their hard-earned knowledge. Whether as part of paid employment, pure training or pre-professional affiliation, these people often shared the very best of their practice with me, which they really didn't have to do. A few words of gratitude, a thank-you note–even a small gift–can mean a lot to a tutor and may well encourage them to keep passing on their knowledge.

As you progress, make sure to develop international experience, if you can afford it. Visit different private practices or rehabilitation centres in different countries to pick up new experiences within the private and public sectors. Work abroad for an extended period, making sure you visit and experience different places and don't stay put in one spot.

## Once you feel ready and comfortable with what you've seen and done–then you will be ready to take the next step forward.

This step can be a full-time or part-time job in a private practice in which you will be able to build up and look after a real client base over time.

The feedback you will receive from your superiors, your practice manager and the clinic's patients will tell you in no uncertain terms how ready you are to deal with and look after your own practice–and client base–in the future.

However brilliant you might be as a trainee or assistant, don't run away with the idea that you 'own' your clients or have any partnership status at the practice. That statement is valid even if you have already become self-employed and are beginning to make significant contributions to the practice.

As a trainee or new graduate, keep in mind that you're a learner; your status is 'professional guest' within the practice. You are not there to make big money since you're not sharing any of the risks of owning the business. You spent nothing to buy the business, nor were you in on building it from scratch; you didn't risk a penny of your precious savings to develop it or maintain it.

You are there to work for the owner, to help them build the practice. In return, you hope to learn as much as you can about what it means to run a private practice so that, one day–sooner rather than later–you'll be able use that experience to set up your own successful practice.

Even if you're offered a permanent position, you should still plan to leave at some point. You have to move on, to keep climbing your learning curve. I believe in being open and honest with your host or employer about it when you've made your decision. And always–always!–leave a trainee period on good terms.

As mentioned earlier, thank your employer and your mentors for devoting their time–even if they ask you to leave. And if that happens, do your best not to show or express resentment. Don't make them feel uncomfortable about asking you to leave, whatever the reason may be. And even if you are somehow entitled to additional compensation, I would personally recommend that you do not demand or accept it. Through the training and guidance you've received and the knowledge you've acquired, you've potentially gained far more than any financial compensation is worth. Hence, think very carefully before taking any action against someone who you may need later for a reference or personal recommendation.

Practitioners, however, are strongly advised through the 'duty of candour' applying to healthcare professionals to take action and not to accept it if there has been any untoward (offensive or inappropriate) activity or behaviour.

---

## Once you've completed your generic physiotherapy and work experience of different types, in different places and with different professionals, you are ready to move on.

---

By now you should have received positive feedback from your supervisors and your clients and therefore you will be ready to move ahead.

In the next chapter, I'll backtrack a little to explore my suggested professional development pathways. By following a similar, yet not necessarily an identical, pathway to mine, you are likely to earn professional trust as an educated and experienced private physiotherapist both from your and clients and your peers. With a private physiotherapy attitude and its nature of looking after private client being key elements, you'll certainly step forward towards your private practice dream!

# 3 – QUALIFICATIONS, QUALIFICATIONS, QUALIFICATIONS

●

## MSKP and MT

The International Federation of Orthopaedic Manipulative Physical Therapists Incorporated (IFOMPT) represents groups of physiotherapists around the world who have completed stringent post-registration/post-graduation specialisation programmes in the field of neuromusculoskeletal disorders. As an umbrella organisation for specialised physiotherapists, IFOMPT actively encourages improved patient management by means of its standards documentation and by actively endorsing evidence-based practice. IFOMPT was formed in 1974 and is a subgroup of World Physiotherapy, with the British Musculoskeletal Association of Chartered Physiotherapists (MACP) being a subdivision of it and its specialist organisation in the UK.

As was previously mentioned, the traditional title of 'Manipulative Physiotherapy', which is also called 'Manual Therapy', was recently changed for British MACP members to 'Musculoskeletal (MSK) Physiotherapy'. I should point out that MSKP, though not including the word 'neuro', still includes professional education, assessment and treatment of the human body's nervous system.

The former professional title was used also in the UK for many years, just like for all IFOMPT members, to denote physiotherapists who had completed a series of relevant courses or a postgraduate degree which made them specialists in clinical reasoning of the human movement system, while also training them in manipulative skills to accelerate treatment outcomes.

In this book, the term MSKP/MT is applied in out-patient departments or sports injuries clinics, whether private or in the public health sector. It also represents an example of an advanced-continual learning pathway which is well aligned with private physiotherapy work and would open you to completely new employment and self-employment opportunities.

---

## Ever since the early days of my physiotherapy education, I've noticed that a very few basic traits could make every physiotherapist much more successful in their work.

---

*One*: the physiotherapist's entire attitude towards their own patients.
*Two*: their attitude towards professional development.
*Three*: the professional skills and knowledge they developed, adopted and followed.

Along with your attitude towards your own patients, your attitude towards professional development is a major component of your career development. Although combining a few professional approaches, you may have noticed that I mainly use MSKP/MT studies and the British MACP as my overall professional umbrella organisation and guidance for my clinical work in regard to the content of this book. This always keeps me up to date, legitimate professionally and as current as possible with the evidence base.

Any investment you make in learning resources, such as time and money spent on professional development, is something you should choose with great care.

Say you want to follow my path and choose MSKP/MT, and your aim is to become an expert, then there are three key areas to improve. The first is clinical reasoning skills (CRS), the second is manual skills, and the third is technological methods. Clinical reasoning takes a long time and often a few years to develop. Yet studying theories and applying manual skills effectively and safely may take a shorter time to allow you to demonstrate reasonable achievement. The same applies to quickly learning to use methods of technology in physiotherapy, including devices such as ultrasound, electrotherapy, variations of shockwave therapy and even other and more advanced methods to come. I trust that you will know what you're doing and that you will be fully qualified to use them effectively and, more than everything, safely.

I'll also explain my views on these treatments in other chapters and suggest how to integrate some of these methods so as to support your practice routine and reputation. I will also explain how I've increased my regular income significantly using these treatments legitimately.

I recommend that you shouldn't give your patients a false impression that you're planning to replace hard manual (hands-on) work by passive machinery treatments or exercise-only treatment methods.

A successful private physiotherapist, whether working in the public sector or privately, cannot function without very powerful CRS. This crucial skill enables you to record appropriate information, such as pain and other signs or symptoms, in order to assess, diagnose and treat the problem—or several problems—effectively.

## Comprehensive examination must be followed by the most accurate possible working diagnosis of the problem and its current sources.

It enables you to prescribe treatments that help your patients overcome their complaint as fast as possible.

Private physiotherapy clients want to see someone fast; once they pay directly or through a private healthcare policy for their treatment, they deserve an appropriate attitude—and they expect to achieve the desired outcome quickly, not only because they're paying for it but also because they're busy. They often seem to have very little time to waste.

Poor clinical reasoning leads to poor diagnosis and selecting the wrong treatment methods. Poor CRS can also risk your patient's health *and* your professional licence.

---

## To my mind, treating patients without a structural examination or clinical process of diagnosis prior to treatment is nothing less than professional negligence.

---

I strongly recommend that you make development of your CRS your very highest priority, using all available means and resources. A good way to improve your CRS is to take a full MSKP/MT or Orthopaedic Manual Therapy (OMT) programme, part-time or full-time, so that you can be recognised officially as a specialist. As mentioned earlier, this is the former 'Manual Therapy' degree or qualification, whether at master's level or on any globally or nationally recognised programme. It takes time, but as it progresses, you will start to operate at a completely different level.

If you wish to be proficient, then, when it comes to achieving this core educational element, I would strongly urge you *not* to try to save yourself money and *not* to cut corners. For a start, a single-weekend course can cost the same as half an entire part-time academic course or qualification over the course of one year. Such courses last between one single day and even five full weekdays and teach just a portion or a single level of an entire professional approach. Students often find they need to pay and repeat the same arrangement several times in order to complete the training and gain a reasonable piece of education which they are able to apply.

Moreover, since almost every physiotherapist ends up doing these common short courses of professional education, if you choose that route, any knowledge you gain will not make you stand out from your peers or colleagues. What's more, these courses are often very condensed and packed with useful knowledge and new relevant skills, yet their actual professional impact and value for money without any follow-up or regular guided practical implementation can be very limited.

In addition to achieving full qualification as an MSKP/MT physiotherapist, you should also read professional books, practise your anatomy knowledge, review pathology and biomechanics, observe others, discuss cases with colleagues–and always think and reflect while you work. Furthermore, a postgraduate degree will advance your research methods and your reading and writing skills, along with every advancement and recognition you achieve at the Master's level and its degree.

Another area to develop is your *manual skills.*

If you look around, you'll notice how different professions compete for or share the same type of client. Some of these professionals apply very poor clinical reasoning, deliver basic services and provide fast 'in and out' treatments–which may be based on treating joints or soft tissue, different types of acupuncture or various massage techniques. There's nothing wrong with this, but as physiotherapists, we need to assess our clients thoroughly and aim to treat their problems more accurately; treatment should be based on systematic examinations and reasoning.

Many different health care practitioners, as well as physiotherapists, practise without a thorough examination and so are unable to explain their treatment process: what they treat and why they treat it. Yet they still do well in business and see many clients every day.

As a physiotherapist, however, you uniquely have the knowledge and background to develop impressive manual skills to effectively set your customers on a speedy course to recovery. Your combined skill set of clinical reasoning harnessed with superb manual skills will also show your clients that you can do everything your competitors can, but the difference is that you provide it under the clinically safe umbrella of your professional title 'physiotherapist'.

A postgraduate degree or advanced qualification in MSKP, the Manual Therapy pathway or any other equivalent programme will qualify you in full to manipulate joints in the human body safely and to elicit very fast physical responses to your treatment. Bear in mind there are other courses and approaches for you to take advantage of, but they may not lead to the national or worldwide professional recognition you should be aiming for. Such recognised titles in the MSKP/MT field are the UK's MACP–or any other official recognition by the IFOMT.

Eventually, once your clinical reasoning has improved and your manual skills are at a satisfactory level, a sound knowledge of the two will allow you to work in the most effective way. Combining clinical reasoning and manual skills also allows you to use your brain and hands together and to save you unnecessary physical strain during your working day.

Once you've made an accurate diagnosis, based on a comprehensive examination, the treatment to progress can be local and specific in order to resolve complaints in a very short time frame and with minimal effort on your part.

In summing up this important section, I want once again to emphasise the tangible benefits of clinical reasoning and manual skills.

## Patients immediately notice your standard of clinical reasoning and manual skills—be they high or low.

They go hand in hand. Therefore, you should work hard to improve them both.

# 4 – ESTABLISHMENT, MANAGEMENT AND MONEY MATTERS

This is a major subject, and there are no clear-cut answers or failsafe procedures because so much is a matter of trial and error–though to stay profitable and solvent, you have only a small margin for error.

Aside from the obvious, such as paying monthly bills, it's crucial to remember that you must make money all of the time, all by yourself.

## You will need to achieve a certain level of income to pay your bills and to pay yourself.

Being self-employed, or being a company owner, means you must work towards managing everything well enough to pay yourself more–to give yourself a better quality of *personal*–as well as professional–life.

The additional calculated risk you take and the longer working hours you put into running a small business will start to influence the type of enquiries you receive and will eventually secure your job and your income.

You now have a number of advantages:

- Nobody can fire you.
- No one can put your growth at risk.

- You can take as much time off as you can afford, and your phone will continue to ring with new requests for treatment, and the money will keep coming in.

Here are two sets of essential pointers to maximising your income. The first set concerns pricing, the second, your skills and how you present your business. Above all…

## Charge prices that you believe reflect your skills and the value of your services.

Do this by ignoring any commonly agreed-upon or perceived 'market prices'. The financial reason for this is to allow you to afford your clinic expenses, to invest in your knowledge, advanced technology and skills, and to pay yourself a decent salary. Make your initial consultation the most expensive and valuable product in your inventory–during the initial session you will evaluate, diagnose and explain unresolved issues, and while starting to treat them you may also cure these diagnosed issues instantly. Hence, your diagnostic skills and experience are your biggest and most attractive and impressive assets. The treatment sessions that follow will be easier and shorter, and you can afford to provide them slightly less expensively than your first time-intensive evaluation. I tend to keep them at the same price so as to always allow my clients to bring up new treatable conditions as the treatment goes along, or to allow for any sessions that have been left unused.

1. Offer an option to purchase a block of four comprehensive sessions with a 10–15% discount if paid in advance. That way, you won't have to deal with awkward situations about payments which can deter

some patients from coming back; situations such as could happen when conditions naturally aggravate or even relapse by the start of some treatments.

    a.   Money has been paid and a follow-up is already in place, which leaves space to continue with your treatment plan. By charging the above-mentioned treatment block of four session, you will also secure income for a very reasonable and well-explained number of sessions.

    b.   Allow clients to transfer full consulting sessions from their purchased block as a gift or a helpful gesture to friends, colleagues, or family members.

    c.   You can also allow patients to share their prepaid block or a single session with others, or to give prepaid blocks to a friend or a loved one—so that these new referred clients might then go on to buy paid sessions of their own.

    d.   Develop a system of routine clinical check-ups to guarantee that clients return regularly and thus secure your income—but make sure to be always straight with clients. They deserve to understand what they routinely pay for.

2.   These sessions should ideally be prepaid for since some clients tend to either forget or cancel appointments if they aren't suffering from pain or other ongoing symptoms.

3.   Aim to have discount offers or the next session or a block of sessions paid in advance. This is not, however, applicable for guaranteed payment from private healthcare providers.

4.   Once you are well established, reconsider your association with certain private health insurances because they often reduce your fees significantly and require invoicing and other time-consuming administration. As part of the policy, some insurances require the

client to pay any excess amount directly to you, payments which are often delayed or even forgotten.

5.  Monitor payments by private health insurance regularly because they can often be delayed due to incorrect invoicing, or they may even be unpaid by mistake.

In addition:

Reduce unnecessary costs in any way you can, such as materials, courses and marketing which aren't suitable for your current stage, needs or the nature of your business.

- Never give your clients the impression of being 'cheap'—that you save money by compromising on quality, health, safety or cleaning standards.
- Monitor your profits and losses along with your cash flow weekly, monthly and yearly.
- Always keep squirrelling as much money away as possible, and never let your business eat away at your personal savings. Your own bank account will always make you feel secure.

## Your Skill Set and Your Business's Image

1.  You should work mostly from one place: your own branded practice.

2.  Allow yourself to work fast during periods when the demand for your services is high—or slow during quieter times—without compromising the quality of your treatment. This is due to the natural fluctuations in demand for treatments, so to reduce the risk of declined enquiries and losing business.

3.  Apply comprehensive examinations, diagnose conditions clearly and use effective treatments so that clients will experience the value of your service if they need to pay more for it.

4.  Use a strong mix of skills from other healthcare disciplines and master them all. This is to ensure your clients are able to get 'one-stop shopping'.

5.  *Add proven and evidence-based technology to your treatment.* Something like shockwave therapy will enable you to add unquestionable value to your treatment session, while charging extra for it legitimately.

6.  This is the place to highlight that any piece of advice or experience in this book about the subject of money will teach you how to earn more of it professionally and legitimately. Therefore, please take all of the information here to heart, as this advice will help you to increase your income and protect it over time

# Private Practice Attitudes

This book is about private practice work, and how to get the best out of it on your own, as a sole practitioner. So, in this section, I'd like to review the unique spirit and requirements for practising this way.

The reality of private practice, small or large, is different from the reality of working in the public health services. Within your own environment and practice territory, you need to operate–and things need to function–in a manner which constantly strives towards what I call 'private practice perfection' or PPP for short.

Organise your personal life however you wish; invest in what you like, neglect what you dislike–but your practice environment is different.

# You need to be your best—mentally and physically—at all times.

You have to display a positive mental attitude. You have to be well presented, clean and groomed, appropriately dressed and exuding the fragrance of a morning shower, not a recent workout.

You have to look professional, look the part. For me it means meeting my clients clean-shaven with a tidy haircut, washed hands, trimmed nails, wearing company-branded work clothes that are spotless and ironed. My female colleagues have similar criteria and standards for how to look supremely professional to meet their patients.

That's on the outside. As for the inside–your mental attitude–you need to be polite and considerate; to smile, to act in a friendly, supportive and positive way at all times.

You cannot arrive late, be grumpy or share negative emotions just because you feel like it. Your attitude must be all about proficiency and making the best presentation of yourself. Remember, you're on show. Everything about your 'private practice attitude', your PPP, is seen and noted by your clients; the way you act directly influences whether future business will come your way. Go into a busy, long-standing private practice; you'll see that the owner and main practitioner will always project a pleasant, positive and trusted character.

However, if you look carefully, you won't necessarily like what you see. A good number of these private clinics rely on low-paid contracts for corporate health work or post-accident cases who appear at their door, who they treat by using either hands-on or hands-off methods, often with a total lack of a personal or professional clinical approach.

We should not be judgemental towards any form of treatment or service or how it is provided in these larger practices. I respect the ways patients are referred and the level of profit these referrals and treatments can generate for any practice in return for safe, professional and honest care. There are many different people who suffer from various problems and pathologies who need and deserve to receive effective treatment. But what you might experience in such a practice as a practitioner might not support the process of developing the type of practice and specific clientele discussed in this book. Early on in your career you may learn and experience great supporting environments, colleagues and patients who you can learn a lot from. However, later on you'll need to carefully select the right places, mentors and even the range of conditions to treat, which prepare you for your specific private practice career this book refers to.

Let's be honest. Most private practitioners' day-to-day treatments can be pretty dull and repetitive, and their practice is built on patients they wouldn't naturally want–or choose–to deal with.

But if *you* can combine a certain attitude with the right fees, you can create *your* favourite daily reality at your practice and in addition treat *your* favourite type of patients.

Part of your aim here should be to filter out people with serious and chronic medical conditions who have undergone unsuccessful orthopaedic procedures. You won't be fully geared up to handle them in your practice, and you will have a slim chance of fully curing them. This is not to say that you should avoid all of them. You need them, and they should always be treated with respect and care in any private practice.

Just make sure they don't drive your business machine. In fact, they rather slow it down since you alone must deal with pretty much every situation or task yourself.

Some examples are manual handling and transfers, direct medical assistance, creating official invoices, written referrals to medical investigations, necessary reports, legal documentation, treating multiple conditions, and so on. You still need to remember, though, that not every patient will be one of your favourites; you may also need to help people who are not lucky enough to have the money to pay for so many treatments.

Some of these patients may also suffer from health conditions, or multi-conditions, which are hard to diagnose and difficult to treat–but you still need to deliver the same standard of care and service.

With the needs and wellness of different patients in mind, I suggest that once you are working alone, you should focus on developing exclusive and higher-end physiotherapy services.

---

## Your credo should be to create your own professional reality.

---

Your approach to people, to yourself and to your professional development–all three of these together–defines your everyday performance and your approach to private practice.

You will soon find yourself communicating perfectly with your clients from the start, creating great rapport and getting most of them better very quickly. Subsequently, you will get yourself well known as one of the best practitioners around, even though the scale of your caseload may not look as large–or be as large–as other practices'.

# Building a Practice with Little or No Money

Unless you receive financial support at the start of your career, you may not have sufficient capital to start up your own practice from scratch–and if you're new to the profession, your novice skills may be an obstacle to providing an optimal level of care.

Therefore, rather than start a business that might limit you professionally and financially, you should instead build up your own client base while working for someone else, or alternatively, rent a room as your own premises on a part-time basis as your practice, which often comes with minimum obligations.

Whilst working for someone else it is unacceptable to steal customers from your employer, or the owner of the practice, while treating their client base. But if someone new comes in, and you begin treating them from the beginning, they may well decide to follow you wherever you go–once you set up on your own.

Customers who arrive through your employer's contact details are not 'your' customers, and so it is unprofessional–perhaps even unethical–to presume they are.

---

## Only customers who you attract independently can be added to your own database or list of contacts.

---

Some would certainly find you and follow you if you own a practice elsewhere, but you should not officially advertise your new upcoming practice to any MEMBER of your employer's client list.

If you work, for example, in a British National Health Service (NHS) organisation, then you might want to collect some key clients and their suitable demographic profile for your future practice, though you must first ask for permission to collect and keep their contact details and store their personal information safely and in accordance with the General Data Protection Regulation (GDPR) guidelines.

Avoid treating these people while you're working for someone else, or if they're still covered by a larger organisation such as the NHS, which is also employing you at the same time. If the rules of your existing contract of employment are strict, you may put your personal reputation at risk. Once you open your own clinic somewhere, even on a part-time basis, that is when it is appropriate to contact clients from your own genuine database in order to let them know where you are and what you are doing.

As this list grows to 200 and more it may well be enough to start up your own business.

In reality, you need roughly 500 happy clients in your database to populate 15–25 weekly slots at an acceptably high fee.

These numbers are valid during the busier months of the year, but you should bear in mind that around Christmas and the summer holidays private health care businesses tend to slow down.

So, you certainly shouldn't plan for your private practice's grand opening during November or December, the slowest months of the year. Instead, use that time to get everything ready–and open the doors for business in January, when people go back to normal life, start to train again and can afford to spend some money and time on treatments.

Renting a room in a gym can be an ideal solution for a start-up. The rent is relatively cheap, and you can get ongoing enquiries through reception and in the actual gym areas. Business may also come directly from personal trainers and people with gym injuries.

However, you first need to make sure that the gym is not part of a large health organisation, because it might require you to become part of its organised referral system. This can lead to an obligation to perform extra administrative tasks, as well as putting the ownership of your client database at risk.

When starting up your own practice within a gym at low cost, you could offer to look after their staff members in return for several very useful benefits or specific arrangements such as:

- Assistance with initial and ongoing marketing
- Using gym facilities with your customers
- Help with purchasing new equipment
- Genuine referrals from personal trainers and in-house fitness class instructors
- Better relationships with everyone in the facility
- Free parking permit if available

- Free gym and sometimes also a swimming pool membership for yourself
- Regular cleaning and maintenance services

To leave your practice at a gym at the right moment, you will need roughly £10,000 to start your own place of practice with your own clients, and by using your own money. The margin of these initial expenses depends on the place you rent or lease, its size and condition, the equipment you decide to buy or lease, your initial marketing strategies, and so on.

Following the steps in this book will enable you to achieve your own practice safely and effectively within the first two to five years of working from a gym or any other facility that features the type of services you will provide.

As long as you don't make any long-term lease commitments to the landlord of some commercial property, you will have the flexibility to move out of your premises. You will always be able to search for, and find, cheaper and more suitable places to work.

# Moving to a Real Practice

The term 'real practice' in this book means a clinic where you're not part of any organisation that can dictate your business type, prices, branding, fees—or one that can limit your access to clients. In your own real clinic, you operate and manage the business exactly the way you want.

**You should be ready to move on and set up your own clinic when you have enough returning clients in your database.**

In other words, when you're able to move independently to a new location, and you know people will travel to see you because you have the unique combination of skills and service they're looking for. This is, of course, on condition that your move doesn't make it too difficult for them to see you, such as limited parking, inconvenient access or distant location.

In the context of financing your move, it would be safer to keep some savings in reserve to finance another move in case your new location doesn't work out, for some reason or other.

The entire set-up should not cost more than £10,000, which is best financed by a bank overdraft arranged in advance so that you will be able to back up this initial investment with your own savings, if necessary, but ideally not have to spend them. I don't recommend that you start a health care business with no back-up savings. Success doesn't happen overnight, and you should factor into your business set-up calculations the possibility of having to recover from an unexpected financial setback. So, play it safe.

Always look for a flexible contract or lease, even if it's more expensive. You don't want to be locked into a place if you run across a better location, or if you decide to expand your practice at relatively short notice. You may also need, or wish, to close the practice due to an opportunity for professional development, or to take a year off.

Therefore, you should stay financially flexible, and leave yourself with the ability to spend some of your savings on closing the practice so you can start up something else or move to a different location.

A long-term lease can limit you at the start and can cost you a lot of money, especially if something goes wrong with the property. Unlike fixing your own flat, a commercial property must be maintained so it is appropriate for business at all times. I've always had positive experiences with flexible terms and conditions, even though sometimes I had to pay extra for my practice to be where I wanted it.

Find a good, trustworthy landlord who can give you a payment scheme that offers you the flexibility to move, if necessary, based on anything between a monthly payment to a payment every two years. Then have the premises fully prepared for your needs and decorated to your tastes–and move in. Since it's unlikely you'll move again for some time–unless you have to–make sure that you're moving to the right place, with the right conditions, on the best terms.

Here are a few crucial tips about moving into your own premises. Like the popular TV series, the secret is 'Location, Location, Location', but there are other things to consider too.

## Location:

- Find a good location, preferably near, but not bang in the middle of a city centre (parking!).
- Ensure you're near a main motorway.
- Check there is free parking or inexpensive meter parking for you and for more than one client.
- Find a place that is pleasant–and safe at the end of the day, after dark.
- Look for a professional and well-maintained business centre.

## Facilities and Comfort for All:

- Aim for a bright space with large windows and as large a treatment room as possible.
- Make sure your place is accessible for everyone: no stairs and has disabled access.
- Have a safe, private and quiet treatment area.
- Are toilet facilities, and a sink, easily available and accessible? Neither you nor your clients should have to go upstairs or downstairs for this. And frequent handwashing is part of being professional.
- Opt for a simple but professional and clean-looking design.

## Money:

- Pre-arrange a sufficient bank overdraft—but aim and plan not to use it.
- Draw up a detailed business plan and a profit and loss sheet to keep track of your finances.
- Option for a nine-to-five in-house receptionist, which means receiving basic reception services from your landlord, such as opening the door, accepting clients, receiving packages, etc. All of these should be provided by an existing receptionist, if there is one if you are operating from a larger business centre. Do not employ one yourself as yet.
- Seek out an affordable rent that also includes bills, mail, cleaning and other office facilities. Look out for any hidden costs or basic service costs that are extra.
- Aim to find somewhere with extra room for an office and storage—but only if this is included and affordable.
- Try to find premises that allow for expansion.
- Renting and Leasing Your Premises

This is a key issue when you plan to open your own business.

---

# Paying for your premises is probably your biggest monthly expense, often much bigger even than the rent or mortgage of your own home.

---

When calculating your monthly practice rental, even though you should always take affordability into consideration, I still believe that if you're not sure where you will be in the next few years, a short-term, flexible solution is better than saving money for a long-term commitment.

As you are now in a position to be very flexible in how much you charge, and how much money you can make each month, the rent you pay must give you the best possible location, in a premises that reflects the quality of your work, that provides a pleasant environment for your clients and you—and, crucially, that allows you to pay the bills and earn enough extra money to save and invest in your skills.

If your rental expenses are as high as £1,000 (plus VAT) per month, which in my experience is rather pricy for renting just a single room, you should always negotiate a couple of months off for committing to a six-month- or year-long tenancy. If your average monthly turnover ranges between £3,000 and £6,000 to start with, then you'll receive good value in return for what you're paying. If the premises are central, accessible and located in a safe and pleasant area, these factors will all add up to make the services you're paying for optimal.

I would never cross the £1,000 threshold; in fact, I would always aim to pay between £500 and £800 per month overall, whether the clinic is completely independent or partly independent, such as renting a small single-treatment room in a health complex, which you might decide to do before moving to your own premises. When I worked under such an arrangement, and when circumstances changed and the host centre evolved into an organisation which could not accommodate me, I had the flexibility to leave and establish my own place, designed for my own needs.

Keep shopping around; you may well find other places with even better offers.

Even when you establish yourself, continue to take advantage of your flexible yet pricy terms so you can search for new and better opportunities.

Though you are unlikely to want to leave your premises too soon—and you may not want to ever—it's still best to have the comfortable option of giving only one or two months' notice should you ever wish to move. After a year, when you can see that everything is working well, you might want to think about a longer-term contract. As a private practice owner, and in a practice that is pretty much dependent on you, flexibility is always the key.

When taking on a long-term lease, be aware that this makes you more responsible for upkeep and maintenance, which means that unexpectedly high expenses can appear out of nowhere.

This just gives you a brief picture of my own experience. I hope it can save you money and lots of hassle in the long term. It can be very useful to ask someone to help you find the right place and help you negotiate the terms and conditions if you're not sure or experienced enough to do so on your own.

# Employing Trainees, Junior Physiotherapists or Senior Physiotherapists

Sharing knowledge and teaching trainees is part of our duty as professionals. If an experienced practitioner doesn't take the time to teach, then future physiotherapists will miss out on a great source of learning to improve.

---

## Taking students or trainees on board is an ongoing cycle that keeps our profession going.

---

This, however, is easier said than done. I have been a trainee myself, and I've taken all sorts of trainees under my own supervision. I like having someone I can teach what I know, but I also try to learn from them at the same time. It brings a new dimension to the practice, and it can be impressive for patients to know students are coming to you as an experienced physiotherapist to learn from you.

Although working with a trainee provides many professional advantages, it has a few drawbacks as well. These drawbacks concern your patients, you (and the trainee), and money and time.

## Patients:

- Some patients don't like a trainee intruding on their privacy.
- Female patients may find it awkward to be treated in the presence of a male trainee, and vice versa.
- A patient can get upset when being treated by a trainee instead of you.

## You (and the Trainee):

- You need to constantly divide your attention between the patient and the trainee, while at the same time focusing on your own role as a caregiver.
- A trainee in the practice on a full-time basis may make it difficult for you to complete your regular administrative tasks and duties.
- Even a graduate physiotherapist with some experience can't be expected to treat your patients as well as you do.
- You might have a falling-out—or they might simply leave and move on, which may lead to a loss of time, money and knowledge invested in training other professionals to do your job.
- This is not to say it's wrong at all to take students or new professionals in or to train them, but it should be well thought through in advance.

## Time and Money:

- It takes time to train and qualify trainees.
- If you bring in a new graduate physiotherapist who is self-employed, you have to supply them with enough work, which is not always possible.

- Paying a full salary to a new graduate physiotherapist you employ full-time can turn out to be uncomfortably expensive for you.

There are, however, some possible solutions.

From my experience with many different trainees and a couple of long-term employees, I would advise you to lay down for yourself strict rules about learning.

## Rule 1

No more than one day of shadowing (or two separate half-days over one week). This pattern can be best if lasts up to a few weeks, if you're comfortable and it suits the practice routine.

## Rule 2

If you are a male practitioner, aim to have female trainees, and vice versa. The reason lies in patient comfort, namely, to avoid two men treating one woman alone, or the other way round, as some men would prefer not to be assessed and treated by two women. This isn't a hard-and-fast rule, but I would strongly advise you to plan and follow this when you have a trainee working alongside you in the practice.

## Rule 3

Do not take on a full-time trainee unless you are *absolutely sure* that he or she is suitable and skilled to treat your clients and that you can afford to pay them once they are fully qualified and ready to join your team. The best way to be sure is to have the trainee prove he or she is profitable for your practice to start with. That means you have to have an additional treatment room to yours (or make yours available at least part-time) for the extra work, and additional paying patients who are perfectly happy to have your trainee as their practitioner. You can offer clients the option to be treated by a trainee under clinical supervision at a discounted rate, or with extra time, or as a supplementary treatment or any other suitable benefit.

## Rule 4

Do not take someone on who is not a qualified physiotherapist or is not working towards becoming one–unless they are a professional in an allied field who you yourself wish to observe at work in return for you training them.

## Rule 5

Set up a defined time period for your trainee to be with you before they even begin.

## Rule 6

An option for very suitable trainees is people studying towards an MSc in MSKP/MT. Their clinical and practical skills and their knowledge and overall experience will often make them ideal for joining you on a part-time basis. You may want to aim for at least one such trainee per calendar year, who is studying towards their MSc in MSKP/MT and gaining membership of the IFOMPT or the British MACP. You will learn a lot from them, just as they will gain lots from you. They are fully qualified physiotherapy practitioners with few years of clinical work experience. You may also get paid some money for training them. Any extra cash they earn for the practice will be beneficial for you too.

I have a bit more to say about employing physiotherapists. First of all, they will hardly ever be able to deliver work in the same way you do. They may be clever people who are great with clients, but a lack of clinical 'mileage' may restrict them.

---

# No graduate, including myself at the time, would be able to handle the front end of a practice without exposing at least some lack of experience.

---

Even if you meet a top graduate who delivers perfect service for your clients and you're capable of paying them, they will often choose to move on towards opening their own practice, to move abroad or to try a different professional job or experience. There is also the slight chance you will fall out with them for some reason, so that will make you choose to let them go. This is based not only on my personal experience but on the experiences of other private physiotherapists whom I interviewed and chatted with before writing this book. You can create a system that is perfectly suitable for taking somebody on board, but both you and your practice need to be well prepared for it.

Going by my own experience, there are more arguments against than in favour when it comes to giving full employment to a trainee when you have a sole-practitioner private practice.

However, you need to make sure you overcome the arguments against and take people on–at least occasionally.

You may want to take on a 'locum' on occasion, that is, another physiotherapist who is as qualified as you are. You would do this so you share knowledge and deliver your experience to others while learning from them yourself. Also, your clients need to accept the fact that you are not always available, whereas your business needs to keep going.

---

## Helping others by training them may bring you great satisfaction, and it will help your business grow even further.

---

On the other hand, your dream may be owning and running a big business–employing additional physiotherapists and more staff. This, however, is beyond the scope of this book; I don't have the experience to advise you on how to build up a business or run a large organisation.

# Managing and Balancing Your Private Practice Finances

Financial management is an extremely important subject which takes time to handle properly in the reality of private practice, so it is appropriate to devote this whole section to it.

First of all, my advice to you is not to mess around with money. Be straight, honest and keep it on track and in the best order possible. Some invoices for services may not be paid on time, or eventually not be paid at all, and so you will need to keep track of them all, to keep losses to your hard-earned income to a minimum. Failing to track the state of invoiced treatments often leads to a big financial hit, especially when dealing with some large private health insurance companies. Always make sure that invoiced treatments have been paid in full as well as any excess amount as the 'client's liability' when it comes to private health insurance policies.

When you first start out you will have many expenses, and some of them are ongoing as well, so this means a smaller tax bill. Take advantage of this situation to invest in your skills and your business at the same time and declare a good portion of it against your taxes.

Although I didn't save much at the start, I've spent years paying smaller amounts in taxes, while paying for and deducting expenses related to achieving the professional career of my dreams. The disadvantage of it all is that I ended up delaying some of my personal goals for a long while. But hey, we're here to become good physiotherapists, aren't we?

At some point you might reach a stage where you will be advised to operate as a limited company, or even discover this option and consider it yourself. It would often depend on your annual turnover, your expenses, assets, pension contribution and any other taxation and professionally calculated factors. Your limited company in that case, and therefore you as the lead practitioner and owner, may eventually end up being eligible to pay lower taxes. Bear in mind, the additional administrative necessities, followed by your accountancy fees and other charges are likely to increase with a limited company in comparison with those of a self-employed practitioner.

You may almost certainly save money in the long run–but administration is more complicated and tracking your finances will be less clear. This may result in a lack of ongoing attention to your current financial picture. Therefore, your careful choice of a highly recommended, supportive and proactive bookkeeper, accountant or accountancy team is crucial. I would choose an accountant as the type of chosen professional here. However, you may pick a qualified bookkeeper or even do it yourself if you wish to, so long as your end-of-year accounts are well presented and in good order for paying your bills and taxes in full and on time.

With everything I've said so far, I'm certainly not qualified to advise professionally on this matter, and you should always seek professional advice before changing your or your business's status. Yet, the best personal experience I can share here with you about the advantages and disadvantages of being self-employed or a limited company is to speak to an independent adviser and study the matter further. You may also find it helpful to speak to a few business owners to learn from their experience.

I've operated as a limited company a number of times in the past. I found it quite difficult to keep up with my finances, maintain administration procedures and, all the while, know my precise current financial state. I found it easier and simpler to operate as self-employed–and I still feel more comfortable and confident this way.

I re-invest any additional income back to myself, into the business, into my tax-deducted pension plan or into business investment funds.

My own research about and my experience with these two business models revealed no difference in my taxes and fees after expenses–and that's value up to achieving a six-figure turnover.

You need to make sure right at the start that your accountant sits down with you and explains everything in detail.

Be proactive and ask as many questions as you need. When dealing with accountancy firms, be sure to be introduced to the individual who will deal with you directly in the long term. You both need to hit it off and get along well.

If you're introduced to a bookkeeper rather than a fully qualified proper accountant, or to someone with whom you're not comfortable, then reconsider using their service. A mistake here can cost you dear: one bad piece of advice from my delegated accountant nearly pushed me into bankruptcy. It took me nearly a year to recover and get back into good financial shape. So be very careful about the firm you get advice from. Dealing with small businesses doesn't mean accountants make smaller decisions or that you should receive a lower quality of service–and your accountant needs to be aware of that too. Find a good accountant, as you will need to make sure everything is tidy and looks good on your financial side if you need to display it. Think of your accounts as your business certificate.

On the other hand, ensure you don't 'overdo' your accounts unnecessarily. Rather than doing it all manually on spreadsheets, you can use affordable or free software. Such software is sometimes added as a free additional benefit through your business banking services. Your accountant will be able to log into it and pull out what they need. But while it's always good to be organised, make sure you aren't so organised that you end up doing work that saves your accountant doing tasks you're already paying them for! Otherwise, at least make sure you have all your receipts organised physically as well as explained and listed electronically and all in good order.

You should also review your income and expenses on a monthly basis in detail before sending them to your accountant. Your bank account's turnover and your sales diary's turnover can be different, so be aware of this too; discuss any major discrepancies with your accountant.

## Make sure you never end the financial year with any form of loss.

You don't want your bank, a lender or a mortgage advisor to look at your final accounts and see that your business is losing money. It doesn't matter if you have lots of money locked away in savings. Your year-end accounts always need to show a positive balance.

## Choose your accountant based on personal recommendations, not someone who has contacted you to market their services.

You need an accountant who is on your side and helps you manage your money and finances throughout the year–not just someone who comes in to tidy up some numbers at the end.

Lastly, I recommend that you explore and eventually adopt an advanced accounting software which would also link to, and integrate with, your practice management software if you use one. This would help manage your finances and keep them in good order through the year and for when the year ends. I've made my own mistake of not using such software sooner, but now I realise that apart from the automation, speed and accuracy in managing my finances it gives, I also have no problem outsourcing major and regular tasks to save me precious time.

Automation within the entire practice and its financial management is an ever-changing and evolving subject which I strongly advise you to research. Search for and then implement desired technology for both your practice management and finances, since the two are always going to go hand in hand.

# Work, Lifestyle and Life Balance

**Working privately, as well as owning and running a private practice, may be one of your professional dreams. It is certainly a worthwhile target for a physiotherapist to have–and it can reward you constantly over the years to come.**

There are so many advantages to working for yourself, owning your own practice, and ensuring that your client base is looked after well. This takes a great deal of responsibility, from both the clinical and financial point of view. You always need to be alert as to whom you treat, where your money comes from and where it goes.

The expenses of your practice are the equivalent of a full-time salary–but remember that you have to pay *yourself* a full salary too. And you need to earn enough money to treat yourself to vacation and recharging time off work.

When you do take some time off and are not working, you still have to pay your bills on top of your holiday expenses.

## Even though you're not earning, the bills don't stop.

When you return to work after two weeks off, for example, you only have half of a working month in which to make up for your lost income, cover your bills and earn your monthly living salary.

You must always budget for your lifestyle. Stay on the positive side of your finances.

Even if you operate as a limited company and pay the lowest corporation taxes, after claiming all of your expenses you will not have much to spend during the first few years. However, a positive financial statement, even on a small margin, reflects healthy business management and points to a great growth potential.

To give you a rough idea, the following table presents an overview of monthly expenses. I've based this on a clinic with a monthly turnover of £10,000. While it may take time for your clinic to generate that £120,000 per year, it's certainly a worthy goal to aim for. There's a column for you to add your own figures. Bear in mind that this chart of private practice income and expenses is only a simplified example, and every number in it can and should be amended according to your own professional and practice reality. It will always get more complicated though, with fixed and variable expenses, unexpected personal or business bills, large one-off or ongoing investments, and so forth.

If you took out a student loan to pay for a first-degree course, you will also have to factor in paying that back. In England and Wales that could cost you as much as £700 per month. Paying back a loan for a postgraduate degree, across the entire UK or in any other country, will cost about the same or even more.

Alternatively, if you don't owe money for nor are currently paying for any education, I suggest you 'play safe' by including a similar amount to pay for any other ongoing business-related loans such as purchasing professional equipment.

| Example of Monthly Expenses: | | Yours to fill in: |
| --- | --- | --- |
| Indemnity insurance and professional memberships | £100 | |
| Pension | £500 | |
| Clinic rent | £800 | |
| Income protection | £80 | |
| Tax and savings | £3000 | |
| Clinic disposables and equipment | £200 | |
| Salary to self | £2,500 | |
| Mobile, Internet, telephone | £100 | |
| Private health insurance | £50 | |

| Example of Monthly Expenses: | | Yours to fill in: |
|---|---|---|
| Charges incurred by accepting Credit/Debit card Arrangement and/or using overdraft facility Business banking charges | £100 | |
| Parking | £50 | |
| Marketing | £200 | |
| Professional courses | £200 | |
| Repaying student loan/ongoing business loan | £700 | |
| Additional sundry expenses | £100 | |
| Business investment saving | £300 | |
| Business emergency savings | £300 | |
| Total expenses: | £9,280 | |
| Net profit after all expenses: | £720 | |

Your salary, savings, taxes and pension are included as expenses because they're taken from the business account. The numbers above represent an established business scenario and demonstrate how much money is coming out of your account, leaving a small profit margin to play with.

The numbers may change for a clinic operating as a limited company rather than you as a sole trading practitioner. Operating your business in such an arrangement as a limited company offers a number of advantages in terms of security for you and your personal assets by separating yourself personally form the actual business. It may also include tax savings advantages and help with your own employment in the business or with employing others legally. Of course, this all depends on the practice's financial situation and appropriate professional advice, based on how much money the clinic generates, and what you actually aim to achieve in regard to financing.

I've operated both ways. Personally, I wouldn't recommend limited company status until you reach a turnover range of £150,000, but as I've just stated, you should make your own decision on it and take the best professional advice.

A turnover of £120,000 is based on treating 25–45 clients per week, at £60–£90 per session. Time for a full consultation can be 60 minutes and 45 minutes for a follow-up. These two types of session may need to be shorter at times, depending on the type of service you deliver, the patient's state and whatever your fee range is. In shorter sessions you can always provide the same level of service, and shorter sessions allow you to increase the number of clients you treat if you need to. Therefore, leave your time per session flexible and don't specify it in any advertising. This strategy would leave you plenty of time and space for personal development and business growth because you'll be able to easily adjust your diary when you need to. So, using the example above, if you manage to increase your annual turnover by as little as 20%, you can improve your overall practice's financial statement tremendously.

You should then plan and act carefully on the financial side as you go along. The financial picture described above is reasonable, though it may fluctuate up and down throughout the year. Like me, you may have to spend a large sum of your own business money at some point or decide to travel professionally or for long-haul holidays–which means you won't be getting paid for a few weeks, but your regular fixed expenses will still need to be. Money to pay your income tax on time would also need to be set aside.

Lastly, by achieving the numbers suggested above, within a very few years of establishing your private practice, you can expect to make a good living and create a better future for you and your family. At the same time, you should have sufficient financial ability to constantly invest in the business and in your skills and to keep them both growing.

Your income is based on a pricing strategy I describe later, where you work approximately 60 hours per week–a figure which includes administration tasks and marketing in addition to giving treatment. The higher your practice fees, the fewer people you need to treat to cover your monthly expenses.

In my view, if you're using your own money and credit or overdraft facilities, then you should avoid buying your own home while you're building your business. Instead, you should first try to establish yourself professionally. It is a huge challenge to use a large portion of your savings—and commit to a long-term mortgage—too early in your physiotherapy career.

I would put owning a home, important as it is, on a lower priority than developing your professional skills, especially when you're likely to move around to continue your studies or because you will need to invest in business tools as well. As I've already recommended, you should put aside in savings the same amount of money you would need to establish your practice. Therefore, it will be available to rescue your business should anything go wrong. A reasonable figure would mount up to £20,000; half of it would go to re-establishing a new practice and the other half to being able to keep paying your taxes and ongoing bills. Beyond your mere business surviving, any failure to maintain your business profitable would have direct consequences on your personal financial circumstances and possibilities. After all, this would all be down to your own choices, priorities, lifestyle, and just pure personal responsibility.

Once your business is established and is generating healthy financial statements, it will be easier to search for a suitable first home to buy—and your bank will be more open to giving you a sufficient mortgage.

If you need to take out a bank loan, make sure you have sufficient savings set aside in case you need to pay it back immediately for any reason.

For you to stay on safer ground, I believe that only once your practice and your patient database begin to generate the kind of numbers we've been talking about can you take your next risk and make a larger financial commitment, such as buying your own home. You will feel much better about your situation, with enough money saved, a profitable practice and a nice place to live as well.

Once your practice is established, you will be able to pay off your mortgage much faster if you wish, using your practice turnover, which no one can limit.

Running a private physiotherapy practice is a challenge but is also a very enjoyable career. It is important to maintain a good work/ life balance.

# Stay interested in your hobbies, exercise well, eat good, healthy food—and look after yourself physically and mentally.

A healthy lifestyle makes it all much easier, professionally and personally. Your goal should not only be to gain skills and build your business. You also have to remember many other important aspects of your life.

At the end of the day, remember you're not serving the business; the business must serve you. Taking care of your personal life is part of acting responsibly towards your clients. Only if you are looking after yourself can you look after your own business clients.

# 5 – PROFESSIONAL AND PERSONAL SKILLS

●

## Working Alone Effectively

For the most part, every physiotherapist works alone because of the one-to-one nature of personal consultation and treatment.

---

**As a private practitioner deciding to run a one-person practice, you will have to work alone with patients and run the business without a boss or workmates.**

---

There are many ways to leverage the income of a one-person practice to grow your business. You might decide to hire another physiotherapist, to outsource tasks not directly related to physiotherapy, or to rent out some of your space to cover some of the practice's expenses. You may also decide to convert your experience into some online product or educational material such as this book that you're currently reading and learning from.

Hence, remember that right now you're not yet attempting to follow the classical approach of trying to expand and growing into a multi-million-pound business or trying to become a creator before you've even established yourself with a valid and unique professional status. Aim just to stay in control of your small practice and to develop great skills to treat people at a high standard.

At this stage you shouldn't worry too much about generating cash flow passively or how the business will work without you in it. You can find out how to invest your extra cash or seek more professional advice on this matter to get these things right, as you progress.

It is crucial that your clients never feel the service they receive and the quality of the treatment you provide are compromised because they sense you are trying to grow your business by servicing more clients than you can handle and not keeping control of your schedule.

Up front, you should make it clear that even though your business is small, it is well run and they are privileged to be seen by you, personally, as an expert, rather than somebody else somewhere else who might be a random member of a larger team. You should always be available to speak to them in person, to reschedule appointments when necessary and to introduce yourself directly to any clients they may refer to you.

From the outset of treatment, you should avoid misunderstandings and build the right kind of trust by explaining that you purposely run your business on a small scale—and this means that during therapy you sometimes need to answer the odd phone call, send a text message to the next patient if you're running late, or pause a session when there's an urgent need to reschedule an appointment for someone. As long as you communicate with your patients about it, there's no obvious disadvantage, and you are unlikely to annoy them.

If you begin to get much busier than you expected, you should look for solutions, such as delaying replies to enquiries, hiring a virtual or a part-time receptionist, setting up an automatic bookings and cancellations system, or working from offices that take phone calls for you when you're with a client.

If you're sure you can afford these solutions, they might help you move your practice forward while letting you serve more clients and deal with existing ones even better.

Stick to the iron rule of answering no more than one phone call, or sending no more than one text, during a treatment session. Clients will accept two interruptions, but when you're constantly distracted, they will feel they're being ignored and that you're wasting their time.

There are certain clients whose treatment you should never interrupt with distractions–and I'll tell you about them in the section on client management.

---

## Overall, when it comes to working alone and multitasking, being sensitive and responsive to all situations will help you find the right balance.

---

# Social Skills inside the Practice

To be a successful and popular private physiotherapist in your clients' eyes, you don't need to be an extrovert outside your practice.

---

## In fact, it is wise to maintain a separation between your professional life and personal life.

---

In other words, don't socialise or hang out with your patients.

It is fine, however, to accept a one-off invitation for coffee or a lunch meeting, but avoid regular get-togethers until you've finished treatment and your patient has been discharged. I'd generally avoid such meetings altogether, unless such a meeting with a client has a mutual business purpose or if a treatment situation or plan needs to be discussed comfortably and without any rush. In such cases, you should at least aim to make them during the day or right after business hours.

The most important thing about how you conduct yourself socially is how you handle situations inside and outside your practice, such as important business meetings, organised workshops or events that can build your reputation and your business.

As for your social skills in private practice settings, you should aim for a balance: a very professional atmosphere that can still be interactive and fun, for you *and* your clients.

You may feel a need to 'entertain' some of your clients in a professional and informative way by teaching them everything you can about their own body's physical functionality, their injuries and their consequences–as well as showing a conversational interest in their lifestyle and fields of personal interest. You may reveal a few personal details about yourself–though only if they ask. Calculate your answers to such questions carefully and don't volunteer to share.

To 'entertain' in this context means delivering a personal, educational, interesting and curative experience to your client, while aiming to achieve your treatment targets in full.

Your clients must like you as a person, trust you, and become utterly convinced that you are able to help resolve their problems. It has to happen by the end of the first session–not because of who you are, how you look or how you present yourself. It happens because of how you make them feel and how you approached the problem they presented you with. You will need to sense their state of mind, pick up their mood, read their body language–and then you can fully align yourself with their situation, needs and wishes in regard to their current well-being.

The essence of social skills in a physiotherapy set-up, whether private or public, is to understand your client's request for help, follow their story, and deliver your professional service in a manner that best serves their needs.

A session with a client can be a welcome break from an otherwise predictable daily routine. Therefore, your client may view your services as a light at the end of the tunnel: a fast-approaching cure for a long-term and disturbing physical problem. It makes sense to offer a memorable personal and social experience: it leaves your client looking forward to seeing you again.

Needless to say, selling your treatment at the price you choose to set will be much easier if your relationship with your clients is as I describe it in this chapter.

## Be friendly, interested and informative, while remaining structured in your approach.

Remember to listen well to patients and give them hope and inspiration for a better future with their problem and their general health and well-being.

# How to Work Fast in a Crowded Schedule

Part of your professional development should be about learning how to work fast enough to handle a very busy day.

## It's important to know how to provide the best value in the shortest time: to focus on getting the next person through the door.

There is no need to set a time limit for each treatment. Some patients don't care how long their sessions are, *as long as you cure their problem*. The majority of your clients who have enough money to be able to pay you are remarkably busy people. Therefore, it's all the better for them if you can be seen to work efficiently.

Some of your clients who receive treatment as part of their workplace private healthcare policy don't pay you directly, so they are usually less mindful of how long the treatment lasts. In short, you do not always need to justify the money paid with the time you spend with a client.

In my practice, I allocate one hour for initial consultations and 45 minutes for a follow-up–but clients don't necessarily know exactly how long I will spend with them.

It's appropriate at the outset to explain that treatment sessions are not designed around an hourly rate; you are there to sort out their problem, regardless of how much time it takes.

A one-hour consultation is usually sufficient, especially if you don't have a full reception service and everything needs to be done in your treatment room. You'll have enough time to present yourself, interview the client, make a physical assessment and finish with some initial treatment based on your diagnosis. Doing it right will provide motivation to come back and spend more time and money on your services.

A 45-minute follow-up session leaves 30 minutes for re-assessment and treatment, with an extra quarter-hour spare for your patient to get dressed, book the next appointment, pay, and gives you breathing space in case you were running late at the start or finish, or if the client was. It always feels like good value for the money and the best use of their time if you plan time effectively. If your prices are appropriate, you will be able to generate a few hundred, or even a thousand or more pounds per day, depending on how you sell your sessions and manage your marketing and operating system.

With well-developed skills and efficient work methods, you should be able to treat your next client within 15 minutes of finishing with the previous one, if necessary–and you can charge the full price without you or the client feeling short-changed. However, keeping up such a pace may entail finding a larger workspace and engaging trained staff or assistants to work along with you.

I was lucky enough to work under a well-known and genuine private-practice owner, an osteopath clinician. Every day he could see about 40 patients himself for a few minutes each, with help from a few assistants and rotating quickly between several rooms. His diary had twenty additional slots for routine spinal check-ups. He charged about £60 per session at the time, and £25 for spinal check-ups, so it's easy to calculate what this practice made per working day.

On top of that, he also had physiotherapists and other practitioners paying him weekly rent or a percentage of their earnings for some of the space, so his income was not limited only by his own work. His superb full-time practice manager made it all work for years and on a daily basis like a well-oiled machine.

Of course, he was not fully booked every day of the month, and he also chose to take some time off during an average week, but his way of working, his years of complete dedication to his single-practice location–and what he generated in a day– were extraordinary.

There were many rooms in the practice to work from, and he had three or four permanent staff members to support him–and of course his fabulous and dedicated practice manager and staff who kept the place going day to day. Needless to say, his pleasant personality and friendly attitude were truly remarkable, which helped reduce the natural rate of dissatisfaction to the very minimum.

Still, for a single person who sees every patient and treats them manually, this is far beyond any usual capacity for work. His unique take on the traditional way of managing his client base, diary and his entire system is something that will inspire me forever.

As clinicians, our professional views were somewhat different, but there is no doubt that I owe a large part of my professional and personal development to this practice owner, his practice manager and his team, and all the people I engaged with over there at the beginning of my career.

Furthermore, the efficacy, reputation, internal atmosphere and appearance of this practice were simply incredible. His clinic was located in one of the city's very best areas, in safety terms, for people to walk in and out, convenient to access, pleasant and with upmarket surroundings overall, which added value to its heritage and long-term reputation.

For that particular practice, it was never about expanding but just being busy enough. It was about treating people well, to deliver a core signature service along with constantly evolving methods, in the same location by the same and the right people.

Another practitioner I happened to work with, a physiotherapist, was able to competently treat one client every 20 minutes, every day, alone, from seven in the morning to six in the evening, taking hardly any breaks. While it's important to say that, along with some private clients, a great many of his referrals came through state national health benefits and various insurance companies, it was an incredible experience to observe his professional work and his almost artistic management of an extremely busy client base. This was in a small Dutch town, and the owner, despite his busy work schedule, kept what appeared to me a well-balanced family life with plenty of much-needed holidays.

Being a private practice owner, and the lead clinician, you should be able to deal with any number of clients in your daily or weekly diary. You must be prepared to manage an overly busy patient caseload, handle the occasional double-booking mistake, answer the phone and deal with everything else that comes your way without messing up your practice schedule.

At the end of the day, your primary task is to resolve your client's problem. No matter how crowded your diary is, they should all feel valued during treatment, and they should leave feeling their money was well spent.

---

**Clients always appreciate busy practitioners, and your reputation will grow based on it—but they won't forgive you if you place money and profits before their care.**

---

# Safe yet Effective Practice

In physiotherapy, health and safety takes precedence over everything else.

The worst-case scenario is hurting a patient. This can prevent you from practising further, or it may damage your reputation and professional confidence for a while. My intention here is not to scare you off being a private practitioner, but to draw your attention to the consequences of being unaware of, or careless about, your patients' safety.

On the other hand, in order to provide results, you need to constantly take action and to challenge your patients' condition in ways they don't always find pleasant or comfortable. You need to make sure they make progress even if this may cause them a temporary relapse or regression in terms of their expected recovery.

---

**Physiotherapy is not only about reducing pain levels, but also about returning patients to their previous physical function, their previous work capacity and any hobbies they may have given up for the duration.**

---

Of course, this is not to say you need to make them feel worse before they get better! The old phrase 'no pain no gain' is not always applicable. You can identify the severity of the injuries by asking a patient to rate their pain level using the Visual Analogue Scale (VAS) of 0–10. You can also identify the irritability of a patient's condition, which means how quickly they get worse or better again if their symptoms are aggravated. Then you can evaluate the effectiveness of your treatment actions by assessing the initial easing or aggravating factors on the patient's noted symptoms during each session or in between the treatment sessions.

Where prescribed exercises possibly limit the patient's progression, you can always reduce, re-teach or change them. There's always a chance a patient didn't do the exercises for long enough or as frequently as they should–or did not do them at all! You will then have to make the right clinical decision on how to increase the intensity or frequency of the exercises and even the recommended level of current sport or functional activity. You may also want to decide on and apply other forms of training muscles, to mobilise or stabilise joints, or treat neural components, in order to optimise the treatment results, based on an explained progression or regression by your patient.

In my view, as for MSKP/MT, the clinical situation is different and aimed at a more precise level of understanding and application. MSKP/MT, when done skilfully and when it's based on clinical findings, dramatically accelerates your patient's recovery. Some manipulative techniques, however, are traditionally perceived as risky. Therefore, many practitioners prefer to avoid them; they practise 'hands-off' by using therapeutic exercises instead. I'm making no judgement at all here because we should all practice based on our own skills, education, current evidence base, and all the benefits of using them weighed against the safety of our patient. In this regard, I see the great importance of specifically highlighting the benefits of appropriately practised manipulative skills.

Among these techniques are the so-called high-velocity low-amplitude (HVLA) manipulations of the spine, which are also termed 'Grade Five' manipulations. The riskiest amongst them involves using them on the cervical spine, which requires an additional education and a very careful and precise application.

Here you need to be safe–but you should not necessarily avoid these techniques if they are clinically indicated and can contribute to recovery, pain relief and overall physical well-being.

You should build your education and skills towards becoming comfortable with performing all the lower grades of joint and soft-tissue manipulations, as well as carrying out HVLA joint manipulation for the neck, thorax and lumbar spine if you judge they should be used, whilst considering their contraindications.

Hence, part of working fast is being able to apply techniques that help reduce pain, restore normal movement and allow the patient to resume everyday activities quickly and safely.

The fact that some techniques entail a greater degree of risk doesn't mean you should avoid them completely–to be 'too safe' at all costs. They have been researched and well practised worldwide, so they can be part of your professional capabilities.

You need to master them all, or at least study them thoroughly to start with, as they may eventually contribute to speeding up your daily working routine and helping your patients recover faster.

HVLA manipulations can often be gentler and safer than slower, so-called 'safer,' or lower-grades manipulative approaches, which may end up being more forceful, painful and aggressive to an injured human body.

Many practitioners don't even touch the neck, or if they do, only in the safest way they possibly can. Instead of attempting a manual assessment for a sore neck and applying gentle manipulation in a very controlled and clinical manner, they often prefer to prescribe a hands-off method of aggressive self-stretching. This rather passive clinical approach often leads many people to seek a quick fix from other therapists who use manipulative techniques and who will always be happy to treat sore neck joints quickly and at low cost. Their treatments, though, often lack a sufficient clinical process and research background, making them less controlled and therefore possibly less safe and effective in the short and the longer term.

---

**Insufficient clinical process and absence of research background may lead to a less controlled and therefore possibly unsafe and ineffective treatment.**

---

Manipulative therapy is considered safer and therefore more commonly used for the thoracic and lumbar spine regions, whether slow or gentle (Grades 1–4) or the fast HVLA (Grade 5) type. As long as you possess all the training required and take all safety precautions, you should be able to manipulate and treat the entire spine, including the cervical levels, safely and help your clients dramatically.

Once you master the skills of manipulating the entire spine effectively, based on clinical assessment, patients will classify you as a much more capable practitioner. You'll be able to cover their need for what they perceive as a purely skeletal bone and joint treatment, by providing spinal manipulation safely and all together. As your clients will see you as a provider of a complete treatment package, for care which previously was often provided to them separately, you'll become a provider of muscular, neural and skeletal systems, in other words, the entire so-called neuromusculoskeletal system, or just MSK as discussed before. They will prefer to consult you for treating their physical complaints and injuries instead of, and even more often than, going to other manipulative therapists.

Hence, as you develop your skill set further, don't focus exclusively on muscular structures. Expand your knowledge into joint treatments as well. Once your manual treatments combine MSKP/MT with other muscular or exercise-based treatments, the effectiveness and the speed of your services will soar.

Manipulating spinal joints is only one example of an area in which many physiotherapists prefer to stay 'safe'. However, when practising privately, you need to be proactive and carry out the treatment that needs to be done.

Your client may have to endure a sore neck for weeks, develop severe pain from the sciatic nerve, or chronic pain in the lower back, just because you decided to skip an effective and useful treatment method to minimise a risk that wasn't even assessed clinically.

Some other specific MSKP/MT treatment areas such as Neurodynamics, which includes controlled mobilisation of neural tissue, or the less commonly used Visceral Therapy for diagnosing and treating the MSK aspect or sources of dysfunctions within the inner organs, carry a risk of aggravating patient pain. Yet they have been thoroughly researched, or at least so widely used and well taught; they can be safely integrated as part of your physiotherapy practice, should you choose to include them.

Applying them correctly can be done in a gradual and gentle way. Similarly, even the highest and fastest grade of manipulations can be done gently, at an extremely low force and in a very accurate manner.

Do not be afraid to do what has worked over many years for millions of people around the world. Get out of your comfort zone and take actions proactively–but safely–to help your patients.

> # When treating patients, I imagine standing in a courtroom, successfully defending every clinical decision or professional action I took.

Keep studying, and have lots of current research at hand, in order to back up your knowledge and your skills. This will add to your confidence and can be useful when explaining your methods to a patient or to anyone who might enquire.

## Communicative Skills

> # Your ability to communicate will determine how well your practice does, and what sort of atmosphere you will be working in.

In private practice, your financial and professional success are often dictated by your professional behaviour and how you handle particular daily situations at the clinic. This usually requires effective communication with your clients and associates. While you may not want to hire employees, as I suggested earlier, you still need to find facilities that provide the requisite space to deliver services, such as a reception area, helpful and friendly building management, cleaners, maintenance people, and more. You need to treat these people well. If you do, they will support you, help you, and, when needed, fight your corner for you.

For example, if you treat your receptionists well, they will respect you and make sure your clients are comfortable and well-treated. While members of the support staff may not be among your favourite people, it can still be refreshing to see them, independently of your patients, on a daily basis. If the business centre you work from employs them and pays their salary, then you can easily enlist them as your allies–or if you happen to be unhappy with their work or attitude, you can give your input as a paying client at the property to improve things. In other words, setting up your clinic in a large business centre that provides reception services may allow you to run your own business with no employment needs or property responsibilities.

Bear in mind, though, that every patient should be treated and all money-related administration such as payment collection carried out either by you or a qualified associate you've chosen. Furthermore, nobody on the premises should impact you or your clients in a negative way that disturbs your routine.

Never tolerate a poor professional attitude or rude behaviour that may spoil your clients' experience, your service or your ability to serve your clients well.

I've encountered the odd employee or service provider in a business centre or gym where I've rented my practice who did their job poorly and with an unpleasant attitude. They were taking advantage of my pleasant personality and manners to create a disturbance to my business, and purposely sabotaged my ability to practise comfortably and effectively. If I realise in future there's a pattern to such behaviour (rather than a one-off trivial incident), I will never tolerate it. I will have no choice but to act promptly to stop any such stressful disturbance to me, my client or my work performance in general. My point is that you and I, as hard-working business tenants, are in a strong position and we deserve to be treated well, in all meanings of the word—that is, pleasantly and respectfully, in workplaces we're paying to operate from.

Greet every employee in the building in the morning and throughout the day, offer advice if you notice them in pain; give them birthday cards and invite your permanent and part-time staff out for a meal. They will respond with re-invigorated motivation.

I can't emphasise enough the need to be a strong communicator, and, in the physiotherapist–client relationship, keep the following in mind.

Above all, develop an ability to make your clients like you as a person and appreciate your skills. Beyond the joy of treating someone who likes you, a rapport between you as a practitioner and a client directly contributes to your overall treatment success and your client satisfaction even if some of your treatment goals are not fully achieved. This also helps clients to be more than willing to pay your full fee at the end.

There is no one rule to follow to make yourself likeable; it varies from person to person. You can't generalise according to sex and gender, class and background, age and experience. Everyone is different, and your job is to be sensitive to these differences and adjust your communication accordingly.

I can't assure you every client will like us as people or professionally, but they don't necessarily have to like us in order for us to treat them well and for them to respond well to our treatment. But I can give you a few tips.

First, you should express a general interest in how your clients feel and 'experience' their problems. Talk about their fields of interest, the hobby or sport that may have led to the injury. Try to sense if your client's orientation is 'emotional' or 'technical/logical'–and integrate it as one of your interview tools. Overall, and more than anything else, just listen to what they say and let them speak freely whenever they want. People who are suffering from pain and experiencing other related problems love to be listened to.

Western culture categorises certain traits and tendencies as typically male or female, but while there may be some truth to these age-old traditions, it's probably better to take nothing for granted and to treat each person as a unique individual. You probably don't act 'like the book', and there's no reason to believe your clients will necessarily do so either.

Next, make your clients feel totally comfortable and create trust within minutes. Match their body language, gestures, and expressions and take the lead from there. You'll soon see how they open up to you and start to trust you. Your conversational skills need to be sharp–as do your listening skills and gestures, to ensure you understand what they're telling you.

If most of your new clients are word-of-mouth referrals, then half the job is already done. What you need to do, then, is live up to your reputation.

# Solving Physical Problems

You are qualified to resolve physical problems and you should do it quickly, safely and effectively–full stop. This is why your patients come to see you. Why they pay your rather elevated fees.

## If you fail to understand the patients' problems, you may fail to resolve them.

As a result, you will risk your patients' health, risk damaging your reputation and slow your overall progress as a private practitioner.

It is essential that you start solving the problem *during the first session*. In fact, before the first consultation is complete, you've already solved some of their problems by diagnosing and explaining the injury, thereby helping them manage their anxieties and their personal concerns about it.

You should therefore always ask your clients what they want to achieve and continue to compare their progress to their goals as you take notes during therapy. In this way, you can monitor your problem-solving process at all times.

This is very much related to fast clinical reasoning, which I deal with in the next section. Keep in mind that it's your responsibility to assess your patient's problem comprehensively, diagnose it accurately and treat it effectively. This is the only way solve it to the patient's satisfaction.

# Fast Clinical Reasoning

Before you treat your patient, you need to examine their condition and diagnose their problem correctly. How you decide to treat a problem–or multiple problems–is based on your clinical judgement and how well you can explain it to your patient.

Everything that you find, you will need to treat, or at least explain, based on your clinical reasoning process, which needs to be as accurate as possible at all times. You have to think clinically and reflect on the process before, during and after a session.

At the highest levels of sporting performance, athletes may develop their abilities to perform automatically and to trust their previous training and well-developed skills through repetitive actions, functional strengthening and different methods of high-performance training.

In the same way, as a physiotherapy practitioner, you may need to work things out, apply clinical reasoning and take action. Then you will need to think it all through once again, to communicate any new thoughts about the problem, and to execute related actions again if needed. Just like a professional athlete, you will need to practice the clinical stages of each case effectively again and again, until you master this entire process of evaluation, diagnosis and treatment working structure.

This is a process of reflection, re-evaluation of your performance, physical re-assessment of the problems and modification of your treatment accordingly. It needs to be done with the aim of eventually achieving the best clinical outcomes with every patient that you serve.

Therefore, automating your actions for best results as you become more experienced is not appropriate and can lead to bad professional habits which may hinder the effectiveness of your treatment and the recovery progress of your patients.

You have to learn to do this quickly so that you don't waste treatment time, don't make clinical mistakes–or, if you do, you correct them as you go along.

You should never compromise your client's trust by just treating them the exact same way, that is, using the same treatment methods for everyone, without taking their current symptoms, their condition and existing situation into consideration. If you're not sure, then you can share your thoughts with the client, and move to a different part of your plan or treat different areas which you are more confident and surer about.

You can always come back to the unsolved problem in the next session after you've given it some more thought–which also provides the client with a longer recovery time.

As part of your clinical reasoning, you can identify as many comparable signs and symptoms as possible, treat them and retest them to ensure they have improved with the treatment you've provided so far.

'Comparable signs' are problematic elements which you need to treat and measure as you go along. They can be related to several aspects, such as range of motion, muscle strength, pure balance, dynamic active stability or body alignment in motion, type and level of pain, and even the patient's level of understanding of the problem.

Failure to diagnose the problem at the very start does not necessarily prevent you from effectively treating comparable signs or symptoms, such as pain, range of motion, balance and weaknesses.

You can always work on the basis of a preliminary diagnosis that you can alter as you go along, while accumulating more information.

---

## This is all about working on your clinical reasoning skills all the time and getting better and better at them.

---

You will need to grow your knowledge by professionally observing other physiotherapists and have others watch you and offer critical feedback. Clinical reasoning is, therefore, one of the most important professional qualities that you need to master. Being able to do it naturally, and as your assessment or treatment goes along, is of great mutual benefit both to you and the patient.

## Delivering Real Value during Treatments

---

## The real value of a treatment is not something you can measure but something your client will feel, and you will then know yourself when this value is received and perceived.

---

Do not think that 'doing your best' necessarily means you have delivered real and sufficient value to your patient. The real value of your service is when you reach a point in your treatment, whether during your initial assessment or any of your planned follow-ups, where you and your client feel you have earned it.

Such a major highpoint in your treatment process occurs once your client has received the biggest point of value from you, whether during a given session or in the course of the entire process. This realisation of your and your patient's main treatment goals will be a combination of offering a clear explanation of the problem, delivering an effective manipulative treatment, offering professional diagnostic palpation, pain-relieving treatment using advanced technology, or providing soft-tissue release treatment, all followed by specific exercises to strengthen or improve balance between relevant muscles.

This combination should lead to a measurable improvement in your client's comparable signs and symptoms, which are informative and physical measurements that you've initially collected and tried to resolve during the treatment. This clinical combination and dosage of hands-on along with hands-off treatment, in my view and experience, is rarely found.

It makes for a very pleasant treatment for the patient when active methods are combined with passive and relevant hands-on ones, along with accurate manipulative treatment, all related to a bigger picture of addressing clinical findings.

They may feel pampered and spoiled, yet they've remained well informed and physically active all the way through. They will always be surprised by the effectiveness and accuracy of your work and might compare it to other practitioners they've seen before.

Your patient will look forward to your next session and will not mind paying for your service. They will pay you for the pleasure of receiving extraordinary value for money.

# 6 – IMPROVING EVERY PATIENT IMMEDIATELY

●

## Integrating Clinical Approaches into Your Practice

Different clinical approaches serve musculoskeletal physiotherapists worldwide. Some approaches are backed by strong evidence and depth of research to support their effectiveness; other approaches have weaker evidence.

During my years of studying, one approach taught the diagnostic and treatment systems developed by the Australian physiotherapist Geoffrey D. Maitland (1924–2010), also the founder of the Maitland® Approach. Another approach is the one introduced by James Henry Cyriax (1904–1985), a British medical doctor known for introducing the field of orthopaedic medicine to the physiotherapy profession. These clinical approaches formed the fundamental pillars of physiotherapy education and practice in several Western countries such as the UK, Holland and Israel. They developed and reinforced their work with research, in order to support its clinical effectiveness with a continually growing base of evidence.

An additional practised system called Applied Kinesiology (AK) is based on equally old principles and methodology. It is practised and taught by medical doctors, neurologists and physiotherapists worldwide, claims to effectively diagnose structural, chemical and mental ailments, but so far lacks a robust level of research base and academic acceptance.

AK combines manual muscle testing (MMT) with advanced application of manipulative therapies based on detailed anatomy and human biomechanics. Although there's a lack of a researched evidence base so far, the structural aspect of AK can be taught and explained to practitioners and patients in simplified clinical, biomechanical, anatomical and functional terms.

AK, Maitland's and Cyriax's methodologies can all be called 'clinical' because they test and measure improvements in terms of physical signs and symptoms such as pain, range of motion, muscular control, and strength, as well as level of functionality challenging general or more specific daily-life activities. My aim has been to practise them all, by combining evidence-based approaches with those that, though somewhat less researched, still have good enough clinical explanations.

Studying and then implementing the best of several researched approaches, along with applicable and well-explained ones such as AK can produce an accurate examination with highly effective treatment results. They all share similar professional foundations that often overlap and complement each other.

## The ability to understand, combine and apply researched and clinical hands-on approaches can be a more effective and safer practice for us all to follow.

While you're using combined practical, clinical and researched approaches, you need to adopt the subjective and objective findings from the initial consultation as guidelines for measuring improvement not only later on in the treatment–but also by measuring sampled progress during the very first consulting session. You should test the outcome of treatment methods by continually monitoring them, correcting them and amending them–or keeping them the same–based on the initially assessed comparable signs and symptoms. Doing this is a major factor in achieving rapid clinical progress and therefore overall improvement.

Mastering combined MSKP/MT approaches, both clinically and practically, on top of your basic physiotherapy knowledge leaves less margin for making clinical errors. Using these approaches, your ability to assess physical ailments accurately and to treat them effectively can increase dramatically.

While performing an initial consultation I strongly advise you to demonstrate improvement by using small treatment samples, right after collecting the objective elements. Of course, you must use your judgement about the severity of pain and the irritability of the patient's symptoms, along with considering the type and source of experienced pain and its mechanism.

The presentation of medical hazards, or the so-called 'Red' flags, also need to be taken into account when starting to treat a patient, especially when higher grades (4-5) of spinal manipulations take place.

As a clinical practitioner, you should be able to reduce pain, increase strength level and improve muscle balance and both joint mobility and stability at will.

A combination of MSKP/MT and AK approaches can, therefore, be integrated by employing fundamental elements of explainable assessment and treatment systems, so as to create a stronger level of trust with your patients. Some assessment and treatment tools are very powerful, however; you should not use them on every client all at once.

I therefore advise you to apply the best clinical analysis and intervention with everyone. But if your time is short, then attempt to create immediate results based on your tentative findings and the treatment methods that you've already found effective. Some patients may need instant proof of your skills to gain their trust so you're able to alleviate severe pain levels effectively, or if they require urgent recovery for an upcoming sports event, active summer or winter holiday abroad, or any other important event.

In some cases, people with ongoing problems may be referred to you through the private healthcare insurance provider at their workplace. If they have never seen a therapist before they will naturally assume that their treatment will extend at least through the number of sessions they're entitled to. They won't be expecting a quick fix. So there's no reason for you to try for a one-session cure, to risk running late into your next appointment or exhausting the client to prove your treatments work fast. Alternatively, as some large private healthcare providers may often pay you a reduced fee per session, you might not wish to keep such clients over too many too long sessions.

You need to decide how far to go for each patient during a given session, so you create maximum satisfaction and the best results based on the time you have, affordability, the number of sessions available and the nature of your patient's request for help. There are a few areas in which you can improve your skills to a level that will enable you to get the client better.

As mentioned before, I would recommend a combination of Musculoskeletal Physiotherapy and Manual Therapy (MSKP/MT) along with Applied Kinesiology (AK) which employs manual muscle testing (MMT). MMT contributes to an optimal evaluation and diagnostic process of where physical dysfunctions stem from, prior to applying any manipulative or other treatment methods.

# The Maitland® Approach

An example of MSKP/MT can be based on Maitland's work over his many years of clinical practice, which is part of the basic physiotherapy training in the United Kingdom and some other countries mentioned before.

UK-trained physiotherapists therefore have a common clinical background that creates common practice principles across the profession. In reality, though, many physiotherapy practitioners tend not to follow Maitland's system for diagnosing and treating physical conditions and sports injuries. I believe this is due to the Maitland® Approach, which demands a high level of prerequisite knowledge and understanding of anatomy, which are both necessary to practise this method effectively. Many physiotherapists wouldn't always find the time and space to constantly study and train themselves to this level of clinical practice.

However, different and simpler assessment and treatment approaches may better suit individual different practitioner for various clinical situations. Maitland's approach, used properly, can become a baseline of a practical and accurate system to follow during a clinical examination.

# Cyriax's Orthopaedic Medicine

The Cyriax approach is also a physiotherapy method which is strongly associated with orthopaedic medicine. It focuses on the treatment of soft-tissue lesions around the body with the option of treating them using manual with exercise-based physiotherapy and the option to stimulate recovery by injecting steroidal medications into the affected or injured area. This method has been proven to treat any condition affecting the tendons, ligaments, muscles and bursae, both peripherally and along the cervical, thoracic and lumbar spines of the body. I've experienced Cyriax's approach through studying, implementing and then practising its clinical evaluation methodology during and a few years after my undergraduate studies. I have never implemented injections in my daily practice routine.

# Applied Kinesiology

The third approach, based on the principles of AK, enables you to know how to investigate with a rather high level of accuracy the type of structure involved in a problem. While this method is also based on knowledge of applied anatomy and biomechanics, it uses gentle 'manual provocation' to an involved element such as muscle, joint, ligaments or a nerve, in order to clinically identify relevant anatomical components.

Hence, AK uses MMT to test the tone of indicating and associating muscles within anatomical muscle chains, movement patterns or the interrelationship between specific muscles. The outcome will then indicate the location of the problem and its underlying mechanics so that it can be treated effectively. AK's examination of muscles using MMT can lead you to the right structure, whether it's a joint, ligament, muscle, nerve or even related internal organs. It uses a rather holistic yet still clinical method to assess problems and to treat them both manually, by exercises or functionally.

There are other examination and treatment systems that you can learn, follow and combine in your assessment and treatment, as long as you understand them yourself and are able to explain them to your patient and perform treatments safely.

---

**You need to work accurately, safely and proactively when performing MSKP/MT to accelerate treatment results.**

---

Hence, I can't stress enough the importance of MSKP/MT combined with AK or other closely associated, widely practised and approved clinical methods of your choice. In my view, this provides superior elements to what you need to know prior to starting or advancing a private practice.

Confusing as it may sound, using a mix of approved professional approaches creates the best understanding of physical dysfunctions in human movement and creates a treatment method that helps to accelerate improvement.

The advanced clinical reasoning and evidence of MSKP/MT and AK can also lead to a much safer and comprehensive practice. As for AK techniques, despite being both holistic and also manipulative at times, they are often based on medical, biomechanical and anatomical knowledge.

Therefore, the AK form of practice can be linked to and integrated well into any type of modern physiotherapy. Since AK's origins stem from old versions of orthopaedic medicine and the early versions of various manipulative therapies, it can also act as an additional in-depth background approach to the modern evidence-based and widely accepted MSKP/MT.

I strongly suggest that MSKP/MT, when combined or backed up with the principles of AK, works well as a legitimate combined approach, which complements the practice of Maitland's and Cyriax's approaches as well as other building blocks of modern physiotherapy. It can lift your therapeutic skills to a completely different level and should become an area you build into your practice as your skills progress. During the first ten years of my career, I was lucky enough to be personally mentored by very experienced and skilled private physiotherapists and doctors who were highly specialised in the older and more traditional manual therapies, AK and human movement in general.

Using this background of knowledge and experience, I figured out the shortest pathways to getting my patients better and have shared it here. The methods I mention are only briefly introduced, but they demonstrate the importance of combining accurate methods with holistic ones in your daily practice.

You need to be good at your learned practice. You also need to be unique and rather more clinically advanced than your competitors and fellow practitioners, including other private physiotherapists, chiropractors, osteopaths, sports therapists and masseurs or any other human body professional. Other fellow practitioners often firmly believe or are even completely convinced that they are equally as effective as or even better than a physiotherapist, despite NOT necessarily working to a clinical and methodical structure of practice.

They all need to be respected for their hard work and for providing professional care, of course, but the uniqueness of your practice lies in the accuracy of your work and your ability to create fast progress, all the while explaining and monitoring your findings at every stage of the treatment.

Finally, we can all act as professional colleagues and support each other, share knowledge and grow the profession. Yet, only when all healthcare providers are able to communicate on a similar clinical level, use an accepted evidence base and measure progress using a common clinical language can the healthcare level worldwide move forward.

# Using Exercises Accurately and Effectively

The need for a comprehensive evaluation and the value of having an as accurate as possible understanding of what we are going to treat and how to go about it are undeniable. Yet there is no consensus amongst healthcare disciplines–or even amongst practitioners of the same profession–about methods to achieve optimal results.

There's an ongoing debate about physiotherapy treatment. Should it be manual or exercise-based? Should it include machinery such as electrotherapy, ultrasound, cold laser, extracorporeal focused or radial shockwave, or even the newer technologies? And if so, what devices should be used?

To the best of my knowledge, current research and evidence in physiotherapy has been mostly focused on exercises. Hands-on and manipulative-based therapies tend to be neglected, often because they're considered time-consuming, require manual work and possibly pose risks to both the patient and the practitioner himself if not studied or trained extensively.

Despite its glorious past, manual-therapy courses tend to be expensive–not to mention that they require clinical knowledge and ongoing development of practical skills.

Therefore, it's understandable when large health organisations and educational institutes who train physiotherapists choose to use well researched, safe and easier-to-learn-and-apply exercise therapies.

> ## However, problems with exercise therapies appear once practitioners use them as a general prescription, without clinical explanation and a selective choice to target problems.

There is a strong evidence base for the positive effects of exercise on people's health and well-being. However, for ongoing physical dysfunctions and sports injuries, exercises need to be selected carefully, based on finding the exact muscular involvement in the treated problem to decide if exercises are needed and, crucially, what exercises to prescribe.

To treat injuries, we need to train muscles by stretching them if they are shortened and tight, or to strengthen them if they are elongated and weak. Overall, we need to decide which involved muscles need stretching and which ones need strengthening or reactivation. Stretching weak and elongated muscle components makes them even weaker; exercising muscles that are already at optimal strength may be unnecessary and can shorten and tighten them even more. Here I wish to point out that I don't mean exercising for the sake of getting fitter or exercising to improve sports performance but exercising clinically or therapeutically to resolve physical problems.

Since our aim is to achieve muscular balance and optimal coordination to obtain a stable and well-aligned skeleton, what we need is to find the desired balance rather than disrupt it even more. Performing muscle testing and examining dynamic stability is therefore critical for knowing which muscles need to be exercised in relation to the problem we're treating.

Any list of prescribed exercises has to be based on the measured outcomes of the selected muscles list, which were clinically tested for their strength, length and their contribution to a given problem in terms of a reduced active joints stability.

How to test muscles, which ones to test for every problem and how to exercise each muscle or a group of muscles is beyond the scope of this book. What is important to emphasise is that we should not prescribe exercises randomly but target them specially to every condition, dysfunction or complaint that we aim to improve.

# Treating with Technology Devices

The need for comprehensive evaluation, along with the value of understanding as accurately as possible where the sources of physical problems lie, and how best to treat them has already been discussed. Yet the most effective of all the different methods to achieve optimal results is something healthcare professionals constantly debate; hands-on or manipulative treatment, an exercise-based treatment; the use of clinically related technology of machinery such as electrotherapy, ultrasound, laser therapy, shockwave therapy, or even one of the newest, which is the still little-known Extracorporeal Magnetotransduction Therapy (EMTT). Going by my personal experience, to the best of my knowledge both the evidence base in support of and the popularity of electrotherapy machine-based treatment have declined dramatically over the years. Throughout my studies and career, I've seen a pattern of old treatment devices being set aside–and even tossed out–in many private practices and public health centres.

It seems clear that the popularity of these devices waned long ago. I think the reason is simply that the effectiveness of integrating technology into daily physiotherapy practice depends largely on how well the therapist understands the theories behind it: knowing what these devices can treat and how they can be used correctly and safely.

> **Despite the aim of becoming proficient in MSKP/ MT, integrating advanced technology into your private practice arsenal keeps you abreast of the latest trends and can add massive value to your overall armoury of treatments and skills.**

Aside from the evidence for the effectiveness of such devices, their passive, comforting and relaxing elements provide an additional benefit: the time spent performing these treatments is not wasted, because you can use it to question the client further, reflect on recent clinical decisions and retest them afterwards.

Lastly, the effect of electrical therapy methods on inflammatory reaction, pain level and muscle tone may in some cases reduce the adverse effects of a physical examination on relapsed and irritable conditions or on very sensitive areas.

Sometimes a client with painful areas or conditions can't bear your touch or endure exercise. This is when hands-free technologies in treatment come into their own, but their proven capacity to enhance natural recovery, optimise inflammatory process and reduce different types of pain should also be considered.

# Finding and Using Cutting-Edge Technology

It's obvious that advances in technology have become an integral part of every aspect of modern life. Yet, though I use some of the most up-to-date electronic devices in my practice, I often feel that in my daily physiotherapy work it's difficult to keep up with innovative technology.

I am always on the lookout for treatments that are well researched, clinically effective and which can be delivered safely through technology–both to assist and to back up my clinical treatment process.

During the 2014 Glasgow Commonwealth Games, where I acted as a physiotherapist, we received what was called an 'Extracorporeal Radial Shockwave Therapy' (ERST) device to try out at the central polyclinic in the athletes' village.

ERST is a non-invasive treatment that works by generating low-energy acoustic wave pulsations which target various acute or chronic injuries through the skin. These shock waves are delivered to a target of damaged tissue to promote the healing process.

When I did some research, I immediately found an extensive and significant evidence base for shockwave treatments in general; for treating athletes, its use demonstrated a very positive effect.

A few years later, when ERST treatment passed the British NHS's evidence-base criteria, I decided to purchase this rather expensive technology. By then it had also been shown by the British National Institute for Health and Care Excellence (NICE) guidelines to be an effective and safe treatment method for several commonly treated conditions.

In my own practice, this particular shockwave therapy immediately had a positive effect with clients, helping to reduce the number of treatments and shorten overall recovery time. Most private health insurance companies have since accepted shockwave and classified it as a 'surgically related treatment' due to its ability to often replace and prevent surgical procedures, which means that I'm paid an increased rate, sometimes nearly double their standard fees–while mostly allocating less treatment time and less physical effort per treatment.

It took me just one year to recover the entire cost of the ERST device–an incredible return for such a large investment. I'd expected it to take much longer.

The company then offered me a trial of their newer 'Focused Shockwave' technology, or extracorporeal focused shockwave therapy (EFST): shocks to the treated area that were generated electromagnetically in a much more focused and deeper pattern. Not surprisingly, this new and more advanced device was more expensive than the previous one: it cost nearly three times as much.

I decided to try it out. As before, I used this new focused shockwave treatment in combination with my clinical reasoning approach, followed by manual and exercise-based treatments.

The effect was revolutionary! It was like the difference between flying in a single-engine prop plane and a Learjet.

I felt completely comfortable with increasing my prices by about 25%, knowing that treatment time was likely to be cut by half. Furthermore, using this new device added an immediate clinical effect when I needed to test or demonstrate improvement of symptoms, with no risk of aggravating clients.

The shockwaves in EFST differed from the earlier ERST in their physical properties and mode of generation. This technique is more advanced, with greater magnitude in the standard parameters such as pressure amplitude, pulse duration and impact. It can also achieve increased therapeutic tissue penetration depths.

I've since integrated EFST to treat:

- acute injuries in elite athletes
- joint arthritis
- bone fractures (subject to age, stage of recovery and other factors)
- stress fractures
- lateral epicondylitis (tennis elbow)
- medial epicondylitis (golfer's elbow)

- shin splints
- osteitis pubis
- groin pain
- Achilles tendon pain
- tibialis posterior tendon syndrome
- medial tibial stress syndrome
- Haglund's deformity
- peroneal tendonitis
- posterior tibialis tendinopathy
- ankle ligament sprains
- frozen shoulder
- all other tendinopathies and enthesopathies

The same technology is being used elsewhere in other disciplines to treat urological indications, male impotence of vascular origin wound healing, dermatological aesthetics, and even as treatment of brain tissue for Alzheimer's and Parkinson's diseases.

The very newest technology which I've recently purchased and started to implement is Extracorporeal Magnetotransduction Therapy (EMTT®). This is a non-invasive, evidence- based treatment for acute injuries and more chronic conditions of the musculoskeletal system. The device itself is called a Magnetolith® and has been CE approved (a marking that indicates a product has been assessed by the manufacturer and meets EU safety, health and environmental protection requirements). According to published information and my studies and knowledge so far, EMTT® uses particular parameters of high oscillating frequency of magnetic field energy to regenerate optimal recovery and rehabilitation at a cellular level. It initiates an anti-inflammatory response, reducing pain and optimising inflammatory reactions in affected areas of the body. Among what this technology treats are different variations of lower back pain, symptomatic osteoarthritic joints, long-lasting neural symptoms and inflammation in tendons and joints.

This is an excellent example of where technology assists us with more difficult and complex conditions. Such conditions include very irritable flare-ups of lower back pain, neuropathic pain, degenerative joint pathologies and rheumatic disorders, which manipulative or exercise- based treatments often aren't very effective at treating. Needless to say, purchasing (or hiring) as well as servicing such technology is expensive and wouldn't always suit private clinics in their early stages. It does, however, produce extremely high and new potential financial benefits, which directly correlate to the patient benefit it's capable of providing.

## There's absolutely no shame involved in using advanced and well researched technology for clinical purposes.

While I can't speak for every type of other current technologies available, it is abundantly clear that shockwave therapy, and specifically its focused (EFST) version, as well as EMTT®, are backed by a rapidly growing evidence base, while its clinical effectiveness has been very convincingly displayed. Aside from some discomfort during the actual treatments, it's quick, safe and has no side effects. When you add its profitable features, you could not ask for anything more.

Beyond every clinical benefit I've listed, once these new technologies were fully operational my private practice's profit increased legitimately, ensuring greater financial stability than ever before.

Lastly, we should always keep in mind that technology keeps advancing all the time, with new inventions, versions, and upgrades constantly being released and marketed. Keep searching and learning them thoroughly and pick up the right ones but purchase cautiously. Become well informed of benefits, risk factors, costs of purchase, and ongoing services to suit your needs and your practice's situation.

# Intensified Professional Development

This subject is huge, and one of my favourites, as I am always studying, learning and trying to improve my skills. It is never easy to improve as a physiotherapist and to keep practising 'above the average' in terms of diagnosis accuracy, treatment skills level, practice efficiency and interpersonal communication, all while still remaining an ongoing life-long learner.

I don't say this to brag, but it took me a long time, a lot of effort and lots of money to get the education I needed, to implement it all and yet to keep this process going on and on.

To give you a better idea, during fifteen pre-professional and postgraduate years, I spent approximately £50,000 on professional education. This was not family money or money I borrowed; it was my own, hard-earned cash. As I earned it, I kept spending it to get better at what I was doing.

In this way I slowly but surely became a far better physiotherapist than I would have been if, instead, I had bought my first house too early, spent all my savings on it–and taken long holidays every year.

I do believe in a balanced life, with the exact nature of this balance being our very personal choice, but education takes time and costs money.

---

**Therefore, during the years when you're first starting out, you may find it worthwhile to delay some gratification while you have time, energy and some regular resources to invest in yourself.**

---

After a few years of hard work, I achieved a sufficient academic and professional level to enable me to apply for and be appointed to almost any job I desired in the private sector, as well as to work with top athletes in the UK and abroad. This wasn't a coincidental career process, nor was it due to any promotional pathway, or to being exceptionally talented, but it was the result of a careful plan and execution of professional self-development.

There were three major components to this process: getting better in the eyes of my clients, getting better officially by gaining the right credentials, and getting better in my own professional view.

For typical clients, I need to diagnose and solve problems quickly in the most professional way.

## Clients need to get much better—or fully recover— in an extremely small number of treatments.

To achieve the same level of speed and success for clients with complex conditions required developing into a complete physiotherapist, and to do this I took every professional course available to increase both my hands-on and clinical reasoning skills.

But I found that, as with most physiotherapists, my biggest disadvantage was a lack of knowledge and skills about how to treat joints using manipulative therapies—so this became a priority.

I started to take short and very expensive courses over a period of time—the type that many of my peers were taking—but I found they were not teaching me truly valuable skills, and what I learned didn't stay with me very long after the end of the course. I realised that, in order to become a better overall professional clinician and to apply manipulations effectively, I needed to go back to doing proper studies again; to enhance my diagnostic and clinical reasoning abilities as well as my manual skills. Then, in order to be recognised as an MSKP/MT specialist, I had to apply for a part-time postgraduate university degree.

I knew that what I required to achieve my goal was an MSc in Manual Therapy (now called MSc in Musculoskeletal Physiotherapy). This postgraduate degree gained me membership of a nationwide recognition for a specialist in human movement physiotherapy– membership of the MACP (Manipulation/Musculoskeletal Association of Chartered Physiotherapists).

There are study pathways other than the academic route I followed to learn the practice of MSKP/MT and advance to a high level. However, I highly recommend choosing a long-term course that will give you recognition such as the UK's MACP or any equivalent accreditation of the IFOMPT.

It took me about five years part-time to accomplish this, and it opened up great new opportunities and made me feel much more comfortable about charging higher fees for delivering extremely high-value service for my clients. A similar process will do the same for you–but you can acquire equivalent education in shorter and more affordable ways. However you decide to get there, it will take you far.

Constantly trying to improve is hard work and, like many physiotherapists, l often feel as if I have yet to truly arrive. This should be the same for your development: you shouldn't let yourself feel too good or too comfortable with your professional level and abilities.

## You need to keep learning and advancing your skills further and further.

Part of my own approach, as mentioned before, was studying AK, which I did in association with highly trained doctors from the Manual Therapy Department of Moscow University. I have never in my life seen so much applied knowledge of the human body, combined with superior manual skills, as I observed with these practitioners.

While being trained by them twice a year, over five years, I felt I was able to advance my entire musculoskeletal and manipulative skills as far as I could go.

The training covered the entire human body, and periodically I felt I received so much new knowledge that I had to stop for a while to review what I'd learned and apply it all before I took any more courses. I then started to feel more able to evaluate, diagnose and cure physical problems, all based on choosing the right learning and knowledge resources.

I suggest that you pick your own area of specialty–whether within MSKP/MT or another area–and take a deep dive into it so you can understand the concepts of its original inventors or creators.

You will find that some allied healthcare professionals truly seem to know what they're doing, and it's well worth learning what they can teach, understanding what is suitable for your own progress, and then combining your knowledge with theirs in order to deliver a custom-made treatment for your clients. The knowledge is out there, but you need to find it and use it in its original context, combined with your own experience.

When you finally get to the point when you are well recognised by official bodies, your peers, your clients–in other words, when you feel comfortable within your own practice–don't rest on your laurels. I encourage you to take my advice and never stop learning. Never stop working on improving yourself.

Review notes you took during courses you attended in the past and pick out an approach that you liked and which inspired you. Then seek out more information about it. If you choose to study or specialise in new areas, then choose them very carefully this time.

I recommend that you go for an academic, professional postgraduate degree in your chosen area; in this way your education will be officially recognised nationally or worldwide. Then the ideal way to continue is to find short, focused courses that are specifically related to your chosen specialty.

Such a process of education can take a number of years to complete, but the opportunities it opens for you may be well beyond your imagination.

# 7 – MARKETING YOUR BEST SELF

●

## Your Competition—Who Else Is Out There

A person in pain, who is suffering from a particular dysfunction or injury and needs help, can nowadays choose from many different treatment options.

---

## Physiotherapy is not the only neural, muscular and skeletal healthcare discipline or sports injuries service available.

---

In the UK, as in other countries, you can find osteopaths, chiropractors, sports therapists and a large range of masseurs and alternative therapists, all of whom provide treatments and solutions that may well be similar to what you provide, though at a quicker pace and a cheaper rate than you as a physiotherapist will offer.

People in other healthcare and fitness disciplines or from other backgrounds take part in many different courses to deliver treatment methods within—and sometimes beyond—their knowledge base and core skills. They can market themselves and offer their learned skills to the public legitimately.

Based on my own knowledge and previous collaborations, I'd like to briefly review some parallel disciplines and explain what they can offer in comparison to physiotherapy. My understanding and view of these other professions may be different from others' viewpoints or from the viewpoint of these professionals themselves, and no professional or personal judgement is intended.

It is important to mention that nowadays, when knowledge is so easily available to everyone, there are growing overlaps between state-registered health professional clinicians and the other therapists out there, regardless of their backgrounds and core professions.

I'm not suggesting that any one of the disciplines listed and explained below is better than the others. This is simply an overview of each type of service in general, based on my own knowledge, professional familiarity and past experience with what they offered to my patients and to me personally when I tried them. Bear in mind, too, that all professions are constantly evolving by communicating and sharing knowledge and skills; some practitioners may be more or less skilled, and the professions in different countries might also have different strengths and weaknesses.

## The Chiropractor

The chiropractor performs alternative medicine that emphasises the diagnosis, treatment and prevention of mechanical disorders of the movement system, especially the spine. Chiropractic is based on the concept that most disorders or illnesses affect the body through the spinal nervous system. According to the British Chiropractic Association, chiropractic care uses a range of techniques to reduce pain, improve function and increase mobility, including hands-on manipulation of the spine.

Chiropractors have been in practice worldwide for many years, yet still for some reason most public healthcare organisations such as the NHS consider chiropractic to be a complementary and alternative care. Chiropractors provide a healthcare service which is not yet accredited by the British Health and Care Professions Council (HCPC). In my experience as a physiotherapist who is also trained in MSKP/MT, I've learned that chiropractic treatment mainly involves skeletal manipulative therapy, often in the form of high-velocity low-amplitude (HVLA) manipulations of the spinal joints. The insufficient background of evidence for this type of manipulation, its overall risk and the specific manual skills it requires have tended to discourage studying and using this particular form of essential manipulative therapy tool. Therefore, the majority of chiropractors I've met use this form of spinal manipulation as their primary form of treatment method, as opposed to most physiotherapists, who don't use it all.

The traditional chiropractor assumes that a vertebral subluxation or a spinal joint dysfunction interferes with the body's function, good health and its innate intelligence.

Sometimes called a DO (Doctor of Chiropractic), a chiropractor delivers healthcare to clients by performing spinal manipulation of different types, for the main spinal areas, based on an approach suggesting that the health of the human body is heavily influenced by the position and alignment of the spinal column and every vertebra.

Chiropractic treatment is delivered mostly on the basis of X-ray imagery, often taken at the clinic itself and not through public service radiography or collaboration with consultant radiologists, nor do chiropractors use other imagery tools. Treatment is generally performed with the client fully dressed.

The treatment can be administered in a scheduled routine of follow-up sessions and can be very effective in cases of acute back injuries, but it is also often used as a long-term method to relieve ongoing discomfort rather than also focusing on searching for and resolving the nature or underlying factors of the patient's complaint– whatever causes these might arise from.

This method does not involve soft-tissue and exercise-based therapies, though chiropractors sometimes employ additional helpers or professionals from other disciplines to support them in these areas.

## The Osteopath

According to the British Institute of Osteopathy, osteopaths use a wide variety of gentle hands-on techniques that focus on relieving tension, improving mobility and optimising function, together with providing useful health advice and exercise, if required.

Osteopaths, who are also considered complementary and alternative medical service providers, provide treatments based on the notion that the well-being of an individual depends on their bones, muscles, ligaments and connective tissue all functioning optimally and smoothly together.

The osteopath receives special training in the musculoskeletal system based on the belief that their treatments, consisting primarily of manipulating and stretching a person's muscles, connective tissues and joints, help allow the body to heal itself.

Osteopathy also includes HVLA manipulations, and often does not include strengthening exercises as part of its core treatment, unless an osteopath decides to complement his or her education in this area, or to employ someone else to deliver it professionally.

## The Sports Therapist

According to the Society of Sports Therapists in the UK, a sports therapist performs an aspect of healthcare that is specifically concerned with the prevention of injury and the rehabilitation of the athlete back to optimum levels of function.

They undertake fitness and sports-injury related education and gain treatment skills which aim at treating amateur and professional athletes. They utilise the principles of sport and exercise sciences, incorporating physiological and pathological processes to prepare the participant for training and competition.

The sports therapist completes college or university education to deliver treatment and rehabilitation to athletes and individuals who suffer from so-called 'sports injuries'.

The length and scope of their education and the nature of their practice is more limited than the average physiotherapist, yet sports therapists may still have wider experience in treating sports injuries than some physiotherapists who have not worked extensively in sports or with professional or amateur athletes.

## The Masseur

A masseur is a practitioner who has an education in applying massage therapy, such as deep tissue massage, sports massage, Swedish massage, aromatherapy massage, mayofascial release, and other treatments.

A masseur may be qualified to combine different manual techniques, which, taken all together, target the soft tissue of the human body.

Masseurs deliver treatment based on their knowledge and skills, with their own intuition for appropriate dosage. They may sort out some problems quickly, and often affordably, for individuals who are looking for less clinically related procedures or just to relax and to feel better.

## The Alternative Therapist

In my experience, the alternative therapist is a practitioner who has gone through college or who has undertaken various separate short courses which provide qualifications to treat various ailments by using alternative and holistic methods of care.

Alternative therapy is a rapidly growing trend around the world and is becoming widely accepted, even amongst the strictest health authorities in some modern and Western countries.

The original methods or adaptations of some Eastern medicines, which existed and have been practised for hundreds or even thousands of years, are now officially employed by and accepted by modern Westerns professions.

Therefore, it wouldn't be uncommon these days to see state-registered healthcare professionals who possess and regularly integrate some of the qualifications and skills of alternative therapies.

Despite an increasing wealth of different therapists and practitioners around us, I strongly believe that a physiotherapist who follows the guidelines in this book should not regard any of them as true competitors in treating physically related dysfunctions. Furthermore, modern society is heavily affected by emotional stress and stress-related illnesses, so alternative therapies may find their place in this regard.

---

## Professional competition can be a problem when, on the one hand, you are not sufficiently skilled, or, on the other hand there are not enough clients or associate professionals at your side who have already experienced your skills.

---

Clients should not only see you as a professional with treatment capacities, but also learn to appreciate your personality. Learning to respect you as a person–and as a professional therapist–will build a lifetime of reputation.

Clients will choose you every time they need treatment and will refer people to you who they think you may be able to help.

We are often happy to refer friends, colleagues or family members to someone who helped us and with whom we have had a positive and beneficial experience in the past.

When your abilities are truly able to help people, and when they refer more people to you as a result of your great service, it will gradually set you apart from your professional associates and potential competitors–if, indeed, you regard anyone as such.

You should still bear in mind, though, that being a busy practitioner and having a busy practice doesn't necessarily mean you're skilled enough at what you are doing, or that your private practice is a stable one. There are busy practices around which treat many people, representing a wide range of the general public, though they don't necessarily have what I would refer to as the 'right clientele' for a private solo practitioner.

Your work as a single private physiotherapist can be tiring and quite miserable if you have to deal with certain clients or referrers on your own, clients of the kind that most of your so-called competitors with larger operating business systems, administrative management and staff would commonly treat or accept in their own practices. Such work would often require considerable paperwork for a reduced fee compared to your normal private fees. Some examples that can overwhelm your own practice are: referrers who ask you to produce detailed reports for each client; clients who are unable to pay your fees; demanding individual clients; particular medico-legal cases; clients with very chronic conditions; heavily disabled patients, and ones suffering from background illnesses, who require special facilities that you can't provide; and, finally, some time-consuming occupational health referrals from certain companies who require in-house or home visit services.

# Dealing with Your Competitors

There is an element of uniqueness when it comes to private physiotherapy, but just like any other business, the competition will have no lasting effect when the services you deliver are of a higher quality.

To remain successful in private practice you need to continue planning how to use your limited time effectively for treatments and professional development, as well as working on your abilities to create and maintain the trust of clients.

I've always viewed this as an ongoing race: to stay at the top in terms of the skills and client services you offer, and at the same time stay on top of your bills and maintain your work–life balance.

You can never truly win in this race, or even finish it–but it can be an enjoyable experience with lots of fun along the way. It offers a very satisfying professional life that not many people are privileged to enjoy during or as part of their working career.

Based on the advice in this book, and at a relatively low cost, in a short time you will make so much progress that you may feel you have already won part of this professional race.

One major competitive issue for private physiotherapists relates to other healthcare providers such as sport therapists and alternative therapy providers, who are gradually becoming more accredited and recognised. The type and nature of some of these providers I discussed in the previous section. Yet I wish to hammer home a few points which may help you become a better private practitioner, regardless of the stage you're at in your career or your actual current workplace.

This information will help you get ahead, whether you seek to become a local private physiotherapist or to excel in the public sector.

In order to position yourself above and beyond your competitors, your aim here should be very simple: to do what you do better than everyone else! Forget about marketing, selling and business development, at least for now.

You need to be a superlative physiotherapist and that's it. But let me explain what a good physiotherapist is, in a private practice context.

I see a good physiotherapist as someone who:

- Cares for patients' needs and is always ready to help them all the time.
- Listens and interacts positively, politely and helpfully even if the client is perceived as wrong or challenging.
- Assesses conditions thoroughly and diagnoses conditions as accurately as possible.
- Keeps practice and treatment room clean and tidy.
- Maintains a professional presentation by wearing clean clothes on a clean and groomed body.
- Provides treatment from an arsenal of manual skills.
- Prescribes specific exercises to train individual muscles or muscles groups accurately.

- Is willing to and capable of incorporating technological treatment such as shockwave therapy (ERST/EFST), EMTT or other electrical or technological treatment methods safely and effectively–to assist his patients' recovery.
- Ensures that clients are ready and happy to pay to see them.
- Provides high value and progress in every session to create instant and real client satisfaction.
- Continually improves knowledge and skills, willing to share it with others and to learn from them too.
- Punctual, replies quickly to clients' enquiries, keeps his word, and works with complete integrity.
- There are, of course, other related qualities as I see it, and this book will explain these. For now, I would suggest that you highlight or even cut out and laminate the points above and place them in a very visible position near your work desk.

All of them are priceless when it comes to private practice, so following these rules will help you become one of the strongest competitors in the private healthcare game.

# Word of Mouth

Word of mouth (WOM) is generally understood to be crucial to a business's success, and for private practice WOM, as a buzzword, is seen as increasingly important. However, I have *heard* via WOM of many extremely profitable and successful businesses where the standard of service is poor and the quality of treatment ineffective. I would never recommend them to anyone because I can't stand poor service and lack of personal care in any context, especially when delivered in return for inflated prices.

Large practices may deliver poor or just basic service yet do well, perhaps because of years of maintaining an efficient business system that markets and serves larger groups than a single practitioner's practice. It could also be due to general demand for a quick, affordable and rather basic, sometimes temporary, solution to a problem. However, it is increasingly difficult for a solo healthcare business to survive without positive client recommendations.

The bottom line is that we, as solo practitioners, rely on personal services delivered to specific individuals who form our chosen type of client base.

A person's motivations in seeking and using healthcare services are much more complex than basic requirements like hunger or thirst. Think about how many restaurants and supermarkets people have to choose from–and how little real difference, in terms of what they provide, there actually is between them.

## With healthcare providers, choices are usually informed by much more than a need to fulfil a basic requirement.

Even when a client calls you with an urgent enquiry, if the job you deliver is not appropriate and not of high quality, they will never come back and–even more damaging for the business–they will not recommend you to their peers.

In extreme cases, they may caution others about the 'terrible' service they received from you. I would never subject any business to public 'shaming', but I can't blame or criticise anyone for doing this since I am also very disappointed when I pay good money and then receive what I consider to be poor value and inferior service.

However, despite my disappointment, I would think long and hard about sabotaging the reputation of a small business, knowing that my dissatisfaction may have less to do with actual value than a personal disagreement. But bear in mind that your clients will not necessarily be so forgiving.

When a decent-quality provider increases fees, I don't mind paying the additional amount as long as I receive something unique and better than competitors who are charging so-called market rates. I only feel disappointed if the service falls short. The same goes for your clients.

Rising prices have become a marketing trend, and many marketing gurus assume people will always be prepared to pay any fee. In the healthcare business, if the value does not increase accordingly, then why should anyone pay any more?

My prices are always higher than most of my competitors, but I'm confident my service justifies it. I make sure my clients have no doubts that they receive sufficient value for their money on the one hand and that my services are unique and personally tailored to each and every one of them on the other.

To keep this issue simple, you should not underestimate the power of what your clients think about you and your services. They need to constantly reassure you that your services are up to their standard. You should ask them directly, in the middle of the course of treatment, if their expectations have been met so far.

Specific questionnaires can be useful too, but more than anything else, it's their WOM referrals to you that provide a good indication of personal satisfaction. You may even want to remind them to refer new clients to you if they seem happy with your service.

Here are few ways to create (further) WOM referrals in a quite natural way:

- Send a warm thank-you email or text to express your gratitude for a referral.
- Give a small gift if clients send you a few referrals.
- Provide such clients with an extra session or extra time or service next time you see them.
- Politely ask your clients to refer people to you once their entire treatment is over.

- Ask clients how they are every few months. This will remind them of you.
- Invite them to exclusive workshops and seminars that you would organise for your best clients.
- Provide a professional discount to health and fitness referrers and look after them throughout the year.
- Anything else you can think of that may show your appreciation to the referrer—but that doesn't lower your service's value in their eyes—may be helpful.

Your client needs to love your attitude and must appreciate your skills in order to understand your treatment plan and cooperate with you. This is because a treatment plan is a form of an agreement between the client and physiotherapist. It's about meeting expectations about what you, the physiotherapist, need to do to meet the needs of the client.

As for loyalty to you over time, if and when your clients need further treatment, this will not be an issue. People have a long-term memory when it comes to great services: they will find you. Yet communication with your client base is required to an appropriate extent to keep your clients up to date and to encourage them to see you sooner rather than later.

Communication can retain clients, but it can be costly and, at times, annoying for some of them who remember you and know where you are anyway. So think carefully about it and proceed with caution. On the other hand, some communication may encourage clients who are suffering with a problem to finally make the decision to come and see you.

---

**Invest your best efforts and resources on superb and personal services rather than generic marketing—and you'll find that most, if not all of your clients, will sing your praises.**

---

# Building your Own Client Database

Private physiotherapy practice is basically all about your client database.

A client database is your own growing list of people whom you've treated since you started practising physiotherapy on your own.

These clients, besides being treated and paying for it, also grow your reputation and skills, and have the potential to bring you more and more new clients, but only on condition that you helped them effectively and treated them well.

---

## Growing your own client database can begin very early in your career, even from your graduation time.

---

You can and should take notes on every person you treat, and in this way you can maintain clients' records to use in future marketing.

Eventually, when you decide to set up your own business, you can let them all know the details, and in doing so you can expect to have an active client database on tap. Advertising your private work will then be easy, with appropriate use of particular social media channels.

While still working for someone else, remember, this is not to say that you can steal clients from your first employers, even if you think your employer didn't treat you very well or if you didn't like the terms and conditions of your current employment or self-employment.

You need to find your clients elsewhere and arrange to do so independently. As mentioned before, you can add clients whom you sourced yourself: friends, a colleague from the university, family members and any other viable targets.

A client database of about 500 of your own real, valuable clients can take around two to three years to accumulate–and then it can already provide you with a basic and growing income. This is, of course, if you charge the right prices and set up your practice in the correct way.

If you have a client database of about 500 clients, you should be able to see between 10 and 15 clients in your worst week of the year and 20 to 25 during busier weeks. This weekly number will steadily grow and allow you to make a decent salary to cover your clinic expenses forever. I say 'forever' because it will last as long as you keep your phone number, email and website alive for clients to contact you. Furthermore, this number also depends on how many links to professional associations and close connections to health-related organisations (gym owners, private doctors, orthopaedic surgeons, personal trainers, etc.) you maintain that are easy to support and receive referrals from in return.

There are different approaches to dealing with an existing client database. Some marketing experts advise using it to generate more income when you need it by creating and offering new services–with the hope that some of your clients will get in touch and agree to pay extra for it.

They also advise you to communicate with your clients so they will continue to 'remember' that you and your business still exist.

I see this in a slightly different way. None of the people you have helped are likely to forget you–and if they need you again, they will probably contact you. You just have to make sure that your name and clinic details are available to them and are online.

Timely communication to update your regular clients about changes to and developments in your skills and your practice are important, and they can make a major contribution to your profits. It will also encourage them to contact you much sooner for an ongoing problem they're possibly putting off the treatment for.

There are great marketing experts out there who can guide you through using communication tools, but you will have to invest time and money to apply their advice properly. It is ultimately more important to receive a good return on your investment.

Blogging and sending texts or emails for no particular reason, or with the obvious intent to sell something, can simply annoy some of your clients; it might even be a disincentive to engage with future marketing from you.

This is not to say you shouldn't communicate with people on your client database, but you should pay attention to the how and the why. A quarterly update letter or postcard–even an annual birthday greeting–can be a great marketing tool, though the costs and benefits of such a direct mail exercise should always be weighed in full.

Organising interesting events for your clients can also add real value and may win you and your practice lots of respect–your clients would love meeting you face got face to gain more of your knowledge and experience at no additional cost, to experience a healthy and enriching socialising event, all with no clinical pressure.

I realise I might come across as somewhat negative about regular marketing-related communication with your clients–and my attitude doesn't match the common ideas of door-to-door selling and generic marketing principles. However, you have to consult and go by your own individual experience and personality.

You should try different marketing techniques and strategies, and you may be surprised by the results. But always make sure any marketing actions you choose to take are linked directly with your target market of clients. And even when the market is your client database, ensure that what you're marketing is relevant to most of them. If, for example, you decide to focus your marketing budget on communicating with your existing clients, it would be best to 'test the water' first on a small section of your database, using a small amount of money on it, before spending a large sum and contacting them all at once.

Keep a close eye on your limited budget and make sure that your marketing is not perceived as that of a generic salesperson. On the other hand, you do need to sell your services. As for GDPR, all my clients tick a box that allows me to communicate with them in private or to inform them of any changes (clinic location, holidays, etc.), to send them professional emails personally or to introduce new services of mine that would help them remain active, healthy and fit. Patients' personal details will always remain secure and confidential and will never be shared with other parties unless a client specifically requested me to do so. Therefore, beyond a quarterly or annual letter to all my clients, my ultimate solution is to have a weekly personal communication to 10–20 points of contact a week.

Read over their records, refresh your memory as to what their last problem was and review other relevant information such as recent physical challenges and include some of this information in a text, email or personal letter. Ten points of contact each week will cover 2,000 pieces of communication in less than one year.

That means that you can personally contact everyone on your client database between one and three times per year, depending on the size of your database. At some point, your database will keep growing based only on word-of-mouth recommendations.

This ongoing way of receiving business can be very rewarding and cost-effective: your search for new clients costs you nothing. At some point, while you're registered with major insurance companies and receive their referrals, you will add clients to your client database more regularly, and though they pay very little, if at all, towards their treatment–especially when they're paid through their work policy– they tend to be easier to please and can often act as great ambassadors for you and your practice.

---

**Overall, you are fully responsible for building up the volume and quality of your client base and continuing to communicate with your clients in targeted ways.**

---

Work as hard as you can to please every client coming through your door. Impress them with your personality, your caring attitude, your practice, comprehensive assessment and treatment skills. Connect with every one of them and make sure they look forward to seeing you again in the future. If you built it up correctly, your client database can grow exponentially in a couple of years to provide you with a stable stream of great clients to treat.

# Marketing Tools

There are many different approaches you can take to market your private practice—and all have pluses and minuses. I've taken many marketing actions to promote my practice. Some were extremely profitable at the time, but others proved to be expensive mistakes. They only made me waste my hard-earned money.

There are some of my personal mistakes listed here, along with a starter menu of generic marketing steps which helped me build my practice and gain the clients I wanted to treat. I recommend them all.

### On a person-to-person level...

- building friendly professional relationships with private doctors, private personal trainers, and owners of private gyms and exercise studios;
- offering introductory consultations to professionals who have the potential to refer clients to me;
- keeping to a strict, disciplined 'thank you' policy for referrals (emails, texts, cards, small gifts);
- my own mistake: not to keep initiating and creating even more connections once I was established—it can be time-consuming but totally worth it in the long term!

## As an online presence...

- having the best website possible (but remember to keep it flexible for ongoing changes!)
- creating a clear and up-to-date presentation on Google Businesses and Google Maps;
- designing personal and professional social pages, as well as using an optimised LinkedIn account;
- my own mistake: not constantly investing in one permanent ongoing online presentation—such as a dedicated YouTube or Instagram channel—to make sure I develop myself to become confident and visible online as much as offline;

## Other marketing tools...

- organising an annual direct mail campaign;
- demonstrating my best attitude and skills during every initial consultation with a new client;
- presenting each new client with a clear visual online and 'take-home' model of my professional approach and business process;
- carefully planned and well-presented aftercare and essential 'up-sales' services online and in the physical practice;
- online educational content, which incorporates my core knowledge and is available free during the treatment period and thereafter is subject to payment for use as a separate online educational and preventative tool.

From my understanding and experience of my by now nearly 20 years in private physiotherapy, I would divide private practice marketing into three parts:

## One

The first stage is a building-up: a process that begins before you set up the 'real' practice. This is when you make yourself known privately to other people prior to starting your own business.

At this stage, you can work for someone else and start marketing yourself and your skills using private business cards and providing advice. You can do this as long as you do not in any way 'sabotage' your employer's business to benefit yourself in any way.

## Two

The second stage takes place during the early days of operating your own business, while you build your initial client database and communicate with clients about setting up your business, whether it's a rented space within an existing business or a fully independent private practice.

In this case, you will be able to advertise yourself and your skills in order to attract clients to your new business.

When your small client database of existing or potential clients is developed, it should not be difficult to fill half of your diary and recover your expenses from day one.

## Three

The third stage of your marketing system is continuing to advertise your clinic to existing and new clients when the practice goes into operation.

Here you need to be careful and sensitive with your budget and your means of communication. At this early stage you may not have enough money to invest in mass-scale online or offline campaigns that will guarantee new enquiries.

You have to remember that your clients appreciate you as their practitioner and would be ready and willing to pay for your good services. However, do remember, not all your clients will welcome a regular marketing campaign of emails, texts, and newsletters. As far as they're concerned, you're only there to take care of their body and health when they need it.

Regular marketing campaigns that target all your clients simultaneously can be off-putting; in fact, they may put some people off using your services again. Put yourself in their shoes for a second. How often have you been turned off a good or service through over-marketing?

Some marketing experts, however, would advocate that you should never assume clients feel that way towards your campaigns. My slightly more conservative opinion is that you should not risk losing any long-term clients by sending the wrong generic marketing message just to gain a couple of new enquiries. Also, any intense and pointless social media activity these days is often time-consuming and can lead to a much less controlled public awareness on one hand, while not contributing to your skills or clinical abilities on the other.

## You need to convey a clear message that your clients need you—not you, them!

My word of caution, of course, excludes informative letters about starting up your new business or introducing a new skill or a uniquely new service to established clients. You might also announce things like holidays and availability or send out quarterly greetings to all of your clients with key updates that would benefit them all. Despite my earlier comment on them, modern social media platforms are more suitable for ongoing communication without the feeling of 'annoying' your regular customers unnecessarily, as long as your target clients don't miss out on your messages.

Remember that most people don't even bother answering an email blast; the response rate is generally 1% or so. Still, it's worth doing once or twice a year; even a 1%-response from a few hundred clients can yield a profitable return.

So it's hard to say if existing or even potential clients will respond to communications and whether or not marketing might be perceived as an attempt to sell treatments.

Your clients may or may not accept the fact you need to go out and sell your skills so you can make a living and keep serving them, and therefore it's a delicate choice you have to make about if and how you contact them for marketing purposes.

Overall, I believe the daily practice of your professional attitude and skills is equally as important as traditional or electronic marketing, and perhaps even more effective. Clients are more likely to remember you because they've received exceptional service than from regular group emails or social media posts that you publish.

However, there's only so much a 'static' web-based online presentation can do to attract new clients or retain existing ones. Social media platforms would still offer you new ways to engage with people, and it's well worth your while to learn how to use them effectively. This may increase the chances of new potential clients contacting you in general, but also of existing clients contacting you much sooner, rather than later, when they need you. Viewing you occasionally on their social media accounts, they will also be able to 'tag' you or your business instantly, or they'll remember to refer their friends to you as well.

You need a proactive approach for your private practice, but, more than anything, growing your business is a matter of time and always offering exceptional consistency of service. Remember, to do social media well requires time–and you probably won't want to spend your free time replying to Facebook comments, responding personally or publicly to complaints or participating in discussions while your treatment diary is already full. Lastly, social media has lots of positive and rewarding elements to it. Just remain aware, focused on the clear intention of serving, providing true professional help, and always keep yourself relaxed about it all. If you need to accelerate your business development and get more referrals, one way is by also creating genuine networks. An example of this is helping small organisations and professionally related businesses and their owners in return for recommending you to their clients, which can be a really useful source of new clients.

Sorting out those business owners' injuries can also be an extremely useful way of gaining their trust. I wouldn't recommend free treatments, but it's certainly appropriate to think about a formal incentive to encourage them to see you in person on a regular basis.

Over the years, I have become the main physiotherapy provider for private gyms, trainers, studio owners and private medical doctors; this has made the process of marketing myself and my practice easier.

I do not advise paying for referrals–although I'm not aware that there are any official, legal or professional concerns about doing so. However, it could affect your reputation if circumstances become awkward between you, the client and the referrer. It is not worth this type of risk.

Be very careful when agreeing to any marketing arrangements. Make sure you're completely comfortable working with the referrer, or at least ensure it is ethically safe to do so. Therefore, consult a lawyer or your professional body regulator prior to taking such a marketing action. You can reward a genuine referrer annually through a method of your choice that will clearly show your appreciation. A business lunch or a free workshop can serve this purpose well.

On another important note, the genuine skills and services you're able to provide to clients, friends, colleagues or family members of referrers should always be their biggest reward. Physiotherapy patients are not commodities for trading. When you receive truly appreciated referrals, you still have to spend hard-working time and money and knowledge gained over many years of education to help them effectively. I sometimes need to politely and clearly explain these points to some referrers who kindly, jokingly or even boldly ask me to start rewarding them.

Marketing is a huge area and I recommend you study it and build on what I've discussed here. Just remain aware about generic marketing expenditure if you don't have a strategy or tested knowledge on a particular aspect of it.

Build your own experience based on trying different methods if you think they're appropriate, but keep them on a small and affordable scale. Remember to review the results in order to make a decision about using particular methods that you find effective on a larger scale.

When I first started out, I handed out 3,000 leaflets to local individuals and businesses to help build up my practice, as I thought. From this entire project, however, I received merely two enquiries, the second one two years after the first. It didn't seem, at the time, that this method was effective, though it did help increase awareness of my practice in the area. In the end, it generated enough income to cover the price of the leaflets–and a single enquiry can lead to business growth over time and can deliver new opportunities that you didn't account for initially.

So, keep marketing your practice according to your own understanding and experience, but make sure to build your great reputation as the best practitioner in the eyes of your growing client database as well as creating strong networks among client groups, in large companies and with different health and well-being professionals over time.

## Websites and More about Online Marketing

We live in the age of the internet and information, so sharing is the lifeblood of business.

Yet in your practice no single internet tool, interactive website or smart gadget can cure a client's problem!

Developing your skills is the first and highest priority and has to be prioritised over any external tools. It is, though, very important to consider the balance between your professional skills and the use of internet marketing and websites, since they can consume your entire annual budget and may leave you with nothing to spend to maintain the business, develop your skills–or anything else.

Other areas of expenditure that you must review periodically include marketing and motivational self-development courses of various kinds. Again, from my own experience, while these types of activities can be entertaining and organised attractively, they are run by people who can easily convince you to spend lots of money, even thousands all at once, before you have time to weigh up the benefits and costs.

As interesting and powerful as some tools may sound, the next day you will be left struggling to remember what was presented at these events–and if you do remember, it may well turn out that you lack a sufficient budget and skills to implement what you've learned or to maintain it afterwards!

Internet marketing gurus are often true experts in their field, and what they say can be very useful or, indeed, inspiring. But you have to remember that steps towards implementing even beyond their live or online (free or paid) educational products require investment of more money – hundreds, if not thousands, of pounds in my experience. It will often require you to search for or hire more services, then to keep spending time and money thereafter in order to achieve and maintain sufficient return on such online-business investment.

---

## Recouping £1,000 for a one-off internet marketing investment requires dozens of treatment sessions just to break even.

---

In some cases, this can amount to an entire week of hard work. Even if you do attract clients as the result of an internet marketing campaign, Adwords, SEO, or website development, they all require continual financial maintenance.

Bear in mind that you should already be busy enough just to cover your basic expenses.

You need to develop a clean, professional-looking website that is well maintained, but you will still need to take action and create social media platforms you can choose to use immediately or later as you go and learn more about it. A strong, impactful online presence is extremely important and rewarding financially if done affordably and if it's not overly time-consuming.

Make sure your website can sell your services, and how you do this is something you must think through in advance. Be careful who you find to develop and build your website and choose your internet marketing service provider carefully; some are very cheap to start with but can become expensive for any future needs.

If a designer has built your website and you don't like it or you don't get on with them, it can prove very time-consuming and demanding professionally and personally to get out of this business relationship and start all over again. I was lucky enough at times to deal with a great web designer, so my web platform usually looked good, and it was very reliable at all times. At other times, I didn't choose the right people, or the working relationship with them was costly, counter-productive and didn't progress my business.

As important as choosing a person or company to give your website the look and feel you want is to make sure that people will be able to find you when they look. Search Engine Optimisation (SEO)–elements that boost your visibility in search engines–must be an integral part of your website and be built into the design. It would be difficult to add it in successfully afterwards, even if some SEO expert tells you so.

## Remember the cost of bringing a website online doesn't stop at design, SEO and hosting.

You also have to factor in how to make changes, monitor hits and tweak everything to get better search results. Unless you already have the skills to do all this yourself–I didn't–I recommend that you find experts with whom you have good communication who can implement changes for you and keep things up and running. Bear in mind that a Google search or any internet search for physiotherapy services based on location can be performed accurately and effectively regardless of your website ranking on the entire internet. Optimising a business location with all its details in it can be equally as or even more effective than finding your website itself. A website often acts as a well-presented and interactive business card for people who wish to just find out more about you and your services.

Here are a few hints to help your website and internet marketing:

- Your treatment is personal and so your website has to be about how you can help your clients.
- Your ranking in Google and other search engines doesn't necessarily determine how many new clients will contact you.
- When looking for a physiotherapist, people won't stop on the first page of results; they'll keep going till they find someone they like. So, your page doesn't have to be ranked number one.
- The best web company can be the most expensive and the hardest one to reach when there are problems.
- Being well presented online requires hours of ongoing work; therefore, someone needs to constantly do the job, and it costs money!
- Most people visit your website to look for you already knowing who you are, not to search for somebody to treat them.
- Make sure the website design company you go with was personally recommended to you by someone you trust. Don't choose it based only on online testimonials or because you know the owner.
- If you want to develop an interactive campaign, create temporary landing pages rather than changing your entire website.
- You can sell a product that you have genuinely created to help your client or professional associates.

- Do not advertise or link to a business that never sends you referrals– or at least don't give them any kind of high profile on your website.
- Use Facebook, Instagram, Twitter or any other form of social media if you know how to, but beware of privacy and confidentiality issues.
- Unlike many social media feeds, any YouTube content that you've created and posted will stay there, appear and be watched again and again by different people.
- Study social media tools such as Facebook, Instagram, LinkedIn and YouTube, then integrate them appropriately to your website and internet marketing.

Finally, there are many ways to approach internet marketing or social media when running a private physiotherapy practice. My own experience, however, has taught me that, apart from the initial website cost along with a few further improvements, none of my investments in this area ever gave me a 100% return.

Such investments, however, do have to be made, and some money needs to be spent, but this is not necessarily the best way to earn referrals and develop a strong business.

As physiotherapists, we do not often earn hundreds of pounds per hour or thousands of pounds per day, and therefore we can't pay hundreds or thousands to other people on a regular basis for any job, especially if we don't get reasonable returns on our investments.

Whatever I did in the past with regard to internet marketing, and despite gradually becoming well presented online, I can't say I've ever seen any equivalent returns for it as a result of any given investment in it at the time.

Yet I have to admit that times have changed, and internet and website development tools have as well; they have developed tremendously and have become far simpler to use. It is absolutely worth looking into it and using various social media platforms to gain new clients at a lower cost and in a short time.

# The Slow Periods

Slow periods always happen at some point during the year. The traditional slow periods are from just before Christmas till after New Year and the summer school holidays. Each of them can last four to six weeks.

The slow summer period, at least in the UK, is when many of your regular clients go on holiday with their kids and therefore are spending their time and/or money on leisure rather than therapy–unless they need it urgently. In any case, people have different priorities about using their money–their health and well-being are not always included.

During the winter holidays, no matter how well established your practice is, there will be a major reduction in business. Even if your potential clients have money to spend, they will be busy shopping, celebrating and resting. In addition, they tend not to train hard or take up physical challenges during the holiday season, so they won't feel as many aches and pains during this time of the year.

There's not a lot you can do about these quieter times except have money put aside, and maybe take a nice holiday yourself–since you won't be losing as much revenue anyway. So just wait until it gets better again in January–and it will always get busier as long as you remain open for business.

It's better to make any new major financial investments after the New Year unless your investment requires time, new building work or moving to new premises, in which case the quieter periods are more suitable.

In January, you normally need to submit a tax return and a set of accounts; you may also need to pay fees and taxes. Therefore, make sure you enter this period with enough saved cash in hand so you can pay everything on time.

There are different ways to do well and to sell during the slower months, but these need to be planned in advance in terms of marketing strategies. You may temporarily throw money to the wind if the time of year isn't suitable for your clients to come and see you. However, your previous actions can prove to be fruitful when the time arrives for potential clients to use your services later on, at a time more suitable for them.

Alternatively, you can simply let go a bit and look after your own needs: rest, study something new or just regain some energy for the next year.

---

**If your practice is well established, you should be able to pay your bills and still earn something during the school holidays or festive periods.**

---

I like to sell discounted blocks of treatment during November and December so that, even if people don't physically see me during this period, I will still be paid some money in advance as I move into the slower season.

It can be a good idea to consider sales and special offers to incentivise trade, such as a reduced cost for treatment during this period, so clients who are genuinely either busy or short of cash come back to you before January.

Remember, though, that you should avoid giving the impression you're struggling. Sales should only be considered during quieter periods, and if you offer them, make it quite clear it's for a limited time only.

However, keeping your prices at the same level throughout the entire year will serve you well in the long run. Even during the slow period, I tend to keep my fees just as they are.

You need to make sure that you either continue to work during the festive season or take time off completely, providing you have enough savings to do so. As mentioned before, you too need holidays–and, after you've begun to operate a profitable business, the traditionally slow season is a perfect time to take one.

So be prepared for these slow times. Plan for them by making the right personal and professional decisions with appropriate actions at your practice in advance. Then you will survive them effectively and in the most productive way.

# Value-Based Prices

Unless you find a more effective way to leverage your work, the level you set your prices at will totally influence your ability to earn money to pay yourself, stay on top of your bills and, of course, support your family and dependents.

---

**Prices impact your reputation: people will respect your practice partly because of the prices you charge—and this is always the case as long as you are able to deliver value that reflects those prices.**

---

A slightly more expensive price list may put some people off from seeing you, at least to start with. When it comes to treatment, some people base purchase decisions purely on price.

Regardless of the economic climate, large private health care providers tend to enforce the prices they set, which leads many physiotherapists to reduce their prices. Such prices are often so low that they don't reflect the value of the service at all.

If your treatment helps someone recover and resume normal daily activities, then you have surely delivered some incredible value–and you ought and need to be paid well for it.

The reality is that some major private healthcare and insurance providers often pay physiotherapy practitioners a reduced rate per session, and these fees mostly depend on the length of their sessions or what they perceive as the common market rate.

At some point, I decided to charge above these fees for a single session, and though this has probably meant losing out on some potential clients, the majority of people I see are able and willing to pay my fees for what they receive in return.

Unlike fees through insurance policies, which are often paid long after treatment has ended, my private fees can be paid in full as the treatment progresses, or even at once, by the end of the first consulting session. This helps me to earn the full amount per session– or as a block of four sessions, paid in advance, in return for a discount off the total fee.

The initial block of four treatment sessions enables me to deal effectively with most of my clients' cases, and the price, although discounted, is still far above the market price and always paid in advance.

Since integrating shockwave therapies and more recently EMTT as an additional component of the physiotherapy treatments, I have been able to deliver even higher value for legitimately higher fees.

---

## Combining advanced and researched technologies with clinical and manual skills enabled me to deliver higher value for a well-explained and accepted higher fee.

---

By working fast and accurately I'm usually able to cure or at least improve problems dramatically in two or three sessions. This became much easier with the additional support of focused shockwave (i.e.

EFST) or, later on, EMTT, when its use was indicated, so the fourth treatment is sometimes almost like a paid bonus. The client may show up for it nearly cured, relaxed and very grateful, just for a final review. Sometimes clients who don't need the last session of a block of four decide to use it later on, for a follow-up or a clinical review, keep it in reserve for some future treatment or even pass it on to a friend or family member.

I've found that selling clients blocks of more than four sessions can get them stuck with treatments they might not need, and they may sometimes feel as if I have overcharged or oversold treatments to them.

I don't like it when businesses charge me a higher price than their competitors without delivering better service in return, so I urge you to deliver exceptional and well-explained treatment as a core principle, especially if you decide to charge higher prices.

Another advantage to charging higher prices is your ability to work less for more money. Working less is not about becoming lazy. Rather, it's about dealing with a manageable workload while protecting some spare time to develop your skills, grow your business and carry out administrative tasks within conventional working hours.

The reality is that you can't see more than twelve clients comfortably, by yourself, every day, every week; it is better to earn more money from the number of clients you can see. If you see fewer clients during slow days or weeks, your elevated prices will keep you afloat.

Since this book is hands-on and designed specifically to help you, I'm going to advise you about how much you should charge. But keep an open mind and feel free to make your own decisions, depending on your current situation.

Based on the standards I've advised, the initial consultation should eventually be 30–50% higher than the average private practice rate elsewhere, depending on your practice level, and your years of experience. Your consultation is time-consuming; it's the essence of your knowledge and skills and your whole reputation is very much dependent on its progress and initial outcome.

Similarly, subsequent sessions should also remain in the range of 30–50% over the local average fees, though slightly lower than your initial consultation. If you used that time well, you will have made your subsequent treatments a lot easier and enjoyable for you and your clients. Most of them will start to get much better when they come back to see you.

At my practice, however, I've recently made prices for both initial and subsequent sessions the same so I can always convert them into consultation about a new problem or keep them all transferable, as mentioned earlier. The price should still act as a stimulant for the client to pay for four sessions as a discounted block. The initial block of four sessions should be based on a total of 10–15% discount on initial assessment and three subsequent sessions. Fifteen per cent would make purchasing the whole block a 'no-brainer', but 10% is more than reasonable and leaves you with a larger profit. Aim to include shockwave therapy, preferably the focused (EFST) version, with EMTT if you have it and it's safe or indicated, and charge an additional fee of 20–30% for it so any block already includes the full range of your technologies and is priced accordingly.

Friends and sports clubmates can receive a larger discount of up to 25–50%–though a 50% discount may be too high, especially if it is not truly appreciated. Make sure, though, to restrict offers of this type to very exclusive groups: a few important people, friends or close mates–and state this clearly every time you see one.

I would still try to avoid breaking my guideline prices. Instead, I just deliver better value for my existing prices. Remember, you'd probably never ask for free services or a massive discount from a friend who's a masseur, a personal trainer (PT)–or from the IT guy who is building your website–unless it's part of a mutual exchange of services and time.

An alternative to giving a discount to a selected client is to split sessions into two visits. In this way your price remains the same–but you can provide higher value without officially discounting your services. It often works really well, and your services will be well respected by your friends and other people you wish to serve but not lose you time and business.

I have found that a free 'drop-in' session–a quarter-hour of chatting and getting to know a new client–is very effective, particularly if they enquire about your fees or if they've had previous unsuccessful experiences with other therapists.

A new, happy and ready client is always worth a free pre-treatment detailed chat–but make sure you do not physically assess or treat them during this introductory 'drop-in' session. Never touch anyone or provide direct advice without a completely filled in and signed consent form.

As for home visits, I believe it's best to avoid them; see clients in your clinic if at all possible.

On the other hand, if a client contacts you urgently you may feel you ought to make a home visit–but make sure to add 25–50% to your initial consultation fee. Such sessions take much more time for travelling; sometimes you have to load and unload equipment–and there are greater risk factors at people's houses to consider and try and minimise as well.

Do not hesitate to make home visits if you feel it's necessary. These clients may end up being permanently thankful and will become long-term loyal clients. I've always had great experiences helping people in their homes–but never on a regular basis.

The COVID-19 pandemic–and therefore people's health in general–has also to be taken into consideration when preparing to visit clients who are often older, in poor health and more vulnerable. Discussing the pandemic or advising on this or other health-related matters is beyond my authority and the content of this book. Please seek the most up-to-date information and act safely, in accordance with the official regional or national guidelines.

There are other ways you can earn more money inside your daily practice routine, such as selling particular products or accessories online or offline. Be sure that you trust them all and have tested them as safe and useful to any client with any background condition.

Selling online requires advanced online platforms or investing in stock to sell and post it all through your home or practice. Examples of materials I sell include particular insoles, pain-relieving cream and supplementary devices that are more costly for the client to buy online as an individual item. These items earn the practice a couple of thousand pounds a year as additional revenue, and, at the same time, it's very convenient for the client to buy from me at a very reasonable price so they can start wearing and using the item straightaway.

I would avoid endorsing or selling any product which is consumed orally, or anything that includes known medical or allergenic elements in it, for the simple reason that I have never felt qualified to do so.

You need to ensure your turnover per year is sufficient to pay your bills, invest in your skills and business and pay your salary and some holiday time. Therefore, your practice needs to help you get established financially but always in return for the excellent value that you charge and get paid.

As mentioned, the service you will deliver means charging higher prices than the average rates–and this might lead to losing some potential clients. On the other hand, if the value you deliver is high enough it will help you treat the exact types of people and conditions that you'd like to see coming through your clinic door.

I always increase value according to any rise in my prices and have always been able to explain it to my clients, so they stayed with me and continued to refer people to me. In my years of running my practice, I've had people who struggle to pay my fees, but hardly anybody ever questioned the price tags and the value they received for it or asked for a discount.

# Becoming the Very Best Practitioner–for Your Client

Becoming the very best practitioner in your area is mainly a matter of your clients' judgement, but you should also be very confident about what you do and how you do it.

Each chapter of this book provides guidance about how to get closer to achieving professional greatness. It is best, though, not to think that you actually are 'the best' so that you continue to learn from others and let your clients compliment you.

An important point about physiotherapy is that even a novice physiotherapist knows things you've already forgotten or never knew at all. This is just like preparing food: even a mediocre cook might make a dish that amazes you, even if you're a great cook yourself! Therefore, aim to be amongst the best, but be the best you can without comparing yourself to others.

Measure your achievement in comparison to where you are now and where you'd like to be.

Let other people–and your clients–describe you as 'the best' and as a top physiotherapist; be aware of what you need to change or improve in order to get there and keep improving for them. Also, let the people who use your services judge you professionally, not peers or colleagues who practise the same profession but have never actually tried your services.

## As a physiotherapist, you are not in direct competition with anyone but yourself.

As mentioned before, and despite using the term 'competitors' on purpose, nobody can steal your growing client database since it's composed of how your clients remember the personal experiences they have had with *you*.

Therefore, get to know some colleagues who are private physiotherapists, work together with them, and share your knowledge, skills and business tips–if you can–so that you'll be able to learn even more about how to deliver the best combination of skills and valuable service.

# Protecting Your Reputation

**Apart from your client database, your reputation is your most important asset. You need to protect it at all costs.**

Negative WOM that passes from peer to peer on Facebook, and reviews on Google or on social media sites can damage your reputation beyond repair. They may not necessarily shut your business down, but they might slow it down and lead to a loss of income during your early and very vulnerable days of trading.

One lesson I've learned is to find the right associates to whom I refer some of my best clients on a regular basis. So, start building a network of great professionals who are familiar with you and trust you and your skills so they will continue to recommend people to see you.

However, in some cases, after I established such a cross-referral and recommendation relationship, I realised some professionals were regularly breaching confidentiality. Some of my clients complained. Only then did I become aware of who I was dealing with. Confidentiality must be maintained; it can never be violated.

I found, for example, that some of these professionals I had trusted with my referred clients did things like gossiping during or after a treatment session. They asked too many questions about the client's personal life, asked them out, tried to build a personal or online relationship ... the list goes on and on.

Of course, you can't control how other professionals act or behave— nor should you try—especially those of different disciplines to yours.

In some well-being and fitness disciplines, it is not strictly forbidden and perhaps legitimate to stay well connected and to associate with clients socially so as to encourage business maintenance and growth.

This has hardly ever happened to me before, but if you receive complaints or encounter poor interactions between them and your clients, you might want to reconsider future referrals–not only to physiotherapists but to any bodywork practitioner, personal trainer or any individual professional or organisation whom you might otherwise recommend.

It is your choice how–or if–you wish to interact with your existing clients outside the therapist/client context, but bear in mind that you are a healthcare practitioner. Some types of interaction can generally be perceived and considered as inappropriate.

Therefore, as far as your business and reputation are concerned, you should stop referring clients to someone else if you notice the slightest dishonesty, lack of professional attitude or breach of confidentiality in how they handle their own clients, especially if any of yours are involved.

Having an intimate relationship with a client is another sensitive issue. You can do so–but only after you've completely discharged your client and mentioned it clearly to them as well as placing a discharge stamp or other proof on their notes.

Ideally, you should avoid making close friends or going out on dates with people in your client database. But this doesn't always work out. So just carefully choose the people you see and be very sensible in handling the situation.

I think it's appropriate–and beneficial–to meet a client for coffee or to invite a group of clients for lunch or a business meeting from time to time. The issue is only about the choice of individual, the time, frequency and the type or context of the activity.

If anything happens with a client that you think might harm your reputation, then it's important to act immediately.

First contact the client and apologise sincerely for how they feel, especially if there's a chance you did something wrong or caused some inconvenience. If the incident is definitely not your fault, and it seems that someone may have set out to harm you–or if the situation starts to get out of control–then contact the indemnity department of your professional body to report and discuss the situation in detail.

If the situation is related to treatment or service dissatisfaction, you can offer further sessions at no cost or offer a refund as compensation.

Never assume that such a situation will sort itself out. Be proactive and resolve the problem for your client if further care is needed–and to protect yourself, your name and your reputation.

During my career in private practice, I've been faced with occasional complaints of different kinds, though only two of them escalated beyond my ability to work them out personally with the client, and I had to involve my indemnity insurance. We were able to sort things out with no need for any further legal action.

One issue was a brand-new electrotherapy and ultrasound treatment machine which, because of a faulty component, caused two chemical burns to my client's arm. Needless to say, I felt responsible, even though I wasn't directly at fault. Acting on it immediately led, in the end, to a successful resolution. My client received a sum of insurance money as compensation for some small scars–against confirmation that they would never take any further legal action against me or my practice.

It was a very unpleasant experience, but such things happen, and you should be prepared.

Another case involved an unhappy client who sabotaged my name because of a misunderstanding over a new rate schedule I set up when I moved to new premises and started a new practice. I understood later that this person had recently gone through a personal situation that had contributed to a state of general anger and frustration. I probably lost some clients because I failed to act immediately and appropriately–but in some situations, we just need to accept that we do our best and can't make everybody happy.

Another potential threat to your reputation is being associated with products distributed by multilevel marketing or tapping into professional areas that you're not well qualified in or don't fully understand. Based on my own experience, I recommend avoiding them as much as possible.

I had a short-term association with a few companies which offered products I thought could help my clients' joints and physical performance in a normal, healthy way. It started off great: I sold a lot of the product, managed to help significant numbers of clients, and built up a small professional selling team underneath me. But it wasn't too long before I saw that the marketing system of one of the companies, driven by some ambitious 'supervisors' above me, started to tap into my client database directly and indirectly.

I felt my reputation as a genuine physiotherapist was being compromised, and I couldn't afford to let that happen. The company had an aggressive marketing system and distribution recruitment approach that involved my client database, and this was very wrong for my business at the time.

It wasn't completely wrong for me to go into a multilevel marketing system where attractive products are sold by individual distributors directly to the client. The products were intended to improve my clients' health and well-being. However, I went too far. In the end, I had to choose between my own physiotherapy business and being a salesman for someone else's products.

I liked the sales environment, the change of atmosphere, the lovely people whom I met across the country and also some of the products. But to build up a reputation–and then to protect it–you need to decide what you are professionally and what you are actually best at. Otherwise, you tend to squander your resources and your potential and drift away from who you really are.

In my case, I realised I needed to refocus on practising physiotherapy and selling my own unique skills.

The multilevel marketing system has many detractors, but what I found most troubling was selling products about which I was unsure: their true ingredients, benefits and side effects. These doubts led me to completely stop prescribing orally consumed products of any kind.

In short, if you have your own profession, skills and practice, you don't need a side-line that has no relationship to your core work just to make more money. Be honest with your clients and proactive and creative in your own business; the rest will always follow.

My final word about reputation: nothing attracts more business than your good intentions, integrity and your core professional skills. Don't jump on every bandwagon that promises rapid returns. If you're already successful and have a great name, you can earn good money without gimmicks.

# Should You Expand?

Whether you should expand or not is a major question that I am always dealing with but asking it myself, whether it's right for me, and what form of growth is right for my business. My experience tells me that a single-person private practice still needs to evolve and develop, but that doesn't necessarily mean it has to get physically bigger or expand to a larger business scale.

In fact, I've tried to expand a few times in the past only to realise I didn't enjoy it very much. I had to deal with management issues that were simply not as interesting for me as the clinical ones.

Although it was very satisfying to know I had the personal courage to manage a bigger business, it also lost me some of my financial and personal freedom. I had people on staff to whom I was paying salaries according to their qualifications, but their continued tenure in my business felt wrong while I was struggling to pay myself.

I also had to deal with complaints that didn't come up when I was operating alone. There is no shame in doing it all yourself if you love what you're doing and can handle it well. To be perfectly honest, I like doing my own accounts, tracking invoices, monitoring my practice's financial well-being. It is not unlike the feeling I get in knowing that I am personally responsible for the well-being of my clients.

Some people might describe me as a 'control freak', but this is purely a business question: are you and your business able to expand; are you geared up for it; are you prepared to pull back from the clinical in favour of management tasks?

In reality, running a practice with employees takes you away from your clinical role and makes you a manager rather than a physiotherapist clinician. It's a matter of choice; all options are on the table for changes at all times.

Running a successful private practice and relying on myself gives me the flexibility to work, keep learning, keep travelling and keep on enjoying an active lifestyle and my regular hobbies.

I can enjoy myself without worrying about how my business does when I'm not there.

I keep in touch, so clients are always able to book in; they just wait a week or two and then return to see me when I'm back at work. My holidays normally don't exceed a couple of weeks at a time, so clients may not even notice that I was away or that I took time off unless they contacted me directly, or if I decide to tell them.

Expanding into a bigger practice with more physiotherapists is always a good thing to aim for if this is what you're looking to achieve. But in reality, making money from physiotherapy is harder when you need to pay other people. The average numbers and value of transactions, when converted into your actual earnings after tax and the usual business expenses, are both relatively low. When another physiotherapist joins and is doing your job or sharing it with you, these numbers get even lower on the one hand, with still very limited leverage in it on the other. Such private business requires working physically with the clients on an hourly basis, for an hourly rate.

As your staff are not always adequately trained or skilled, it can often create new problems for you rather than solve old ones. Therefore, based on my experience, the additional practitioner who joins and works besides you will not necessarily make your business more efficient and profitable.

For example, if you operate by yourself with two other experienced and full-time senior physiotherapists, you may need a £300K turnover per annum just to break even–or, if you do make a profit from the practice, it won't be a large one. That £300K figure is achievable, but only with a really smart business plan and a very, very efficient marketing system.

In fact, your initial set-up costs could eat up about one-third of this turnover, and you would need about six full or part-time staff members and a couple of independent marketing contractors to run it all smoothly. I'm sure you may want to challenge this rough figure above, or wonder whether it makes any business sense at all, but I can assure you that any low six-figure income is a perfectly achievable target as a one-man sole business practitioner. When changing from a solo enterprise to a larger business, you would necessarily have to step back and let others deal with new and existing clients while you run the whole operation, which also means doing a lot less clinical work than you'd like. There are many other areas to address when planning a large private practice, but alternatively, if your aim is to practise and deal directly with your clients, then what I've described in this book so far can take you there.

There are still many profitable opportunities you can take advantage of while running your practice and remain a clinician physiotherapist at the same time. If you still love what you're doing, then I would say, why shouldn't you keep doing it?

Some would argue that businesses need to grow and make more and more money, which is true if you wish to run a bigger, potentially saleable organisation and make money this way. This book, however, teaches you how to stay small, at least to start with, while you develop great skills, build a reputation, and make a good living doing what you love as part of keeping a healthy lifestyle and freedom as a physiotherapist.

---

**The reputation you might earn by being rich, famous and powerful has no less value than one that comes from building and owning your own private practice with thousands of adoring and referring clients, making a good living while enjoying it and being proud of what you do.**

---

On the financial side, a solo practice can generate well into the six-figure level of income. If this money is handled responsibly, it can make you very stable financially in your early years. However, you don't have to decide at the beginning whether to be small or large. Start small and grow from there if the situation feels appropriate.

# 8 – CLIENTS:
# YOUR GREATEST ASSET

---●---

## Valued Private Clients

A t the start of this chapter, I wish to state that clients are all regarded equally at all times, without any discrimination of any kind. Once they enter my practice with their request for help, they always will receive the best service I can possibly provide.

Inevitably, you will, at times, be tempted to group clients according to their long-term value and classify them (for yourself) with descriptions like 'reliable', 'fun', 'pleasant', 'pays on time', 'refers others', and so on.

Alternatively, you might classify particular clients as 'tiring', 'energy-draining', 'time-consuming', 'late payers', 'thrifty', 'late for an appointment', and so forth, according to other negative situations you experience when dealing with them.

This is not to say that you can generally tag them as 'valuable' or 'not valuable' clients–not at all. They are obviously all valuable to some extent for you and your practice, but nevertheless some still help you and support your business more than others.

---

### Clients don't need to be tagged in any way or type in order to be classified as highly valued.

---

They only have to be ready to pay for your services as long as you deliver a good return on what they pay.

In general, there are three broad types of client: completely new ones; new clients who come via a recommendation; and returning clients who have seen you before.

Completely new clients haven't seen you before, and no one recommended you. They found you online or through some other form of media, or perhaps received your contact information from a private health insurer. They may be totally new to physiotherapy.

Clients who come because of a recommendation already appreciate your service without ever having seen you. In most cases, providing the above two types of clients with outstanding service may lead to a certain degree of loyalty which might also generate further recommendations and referrals.

Clients who have seen you before and return for more treatment already know who you are and what you offer. They understand what level of service you're going to provide and should be happy about it.

---

## These existing clients are the most important because they come back and tend to regularly refer new clients.

---

You don't need to create mutual trust with them from scratch; it already exists.

A separate group to consider might be friends and people who help you or your business regularly. These people might be colleagues, close friends or distant acquaintances, associate professionals, a mentor of yours, or some other great clients or referrers. These clients are people you want to make sure you serve exceptionally well, and you should consider offering a higher value for the service you provide them with.

A large, permanent discount may also be appropriate if you see these clients or their associates on a regular basis. However, there has to be a clear reason why a discount is offered so as to avoid any misunderstanding when you charge the people they refer to you the full rate.

I would recommend not having too many of them, or to still charge them, just to ensure better value for what they pay or receive from you, as they would often be able to pay for any service they wish to receive.

Free treatments may be given in extremely rare cases: for family members; as a one-off for very close friends or visitors at your home if they need you; and for those attending introductory sessions that may lead to future referrals.

# Dealing with Assumed High-Profile Clients

These clients, who are clearly extremely affluent or even wealthy, sometimes publicly known and famous, and have a good deal of disposable income should be treated no different to any other clients of yours. What they do, who they are or how much money they might have makes no difference to how they should be treated–namely, professionally and confidentially.

Such clients may be chief executives, company owners, property developers, successful small-business owners, artists, actors, producers, or wealthy pensioners–and their spouses or partners.

When they use their private healthcare, which may often pay you reduced rates, you may feel as if you're losing potential income, when you consider how easily they can afford to pay the full price for your services without time-consuming invoicing, forgotten outstanding personal liability excess and typically delayed payments. Therefore, for such reasons and the value of your services, at some point you'll need to decide whether you'd like to keep your provider association with private healthcare providers who cut your fees by far too much.

Bear in mind, though, that these people are often dedicated professionals who haven't always been wealthy, so they can often be quite grounded with realistic expectations about what they're willing to pay.

---

## We should never take anyone's hard-earned money or personal funds for granted or take advantage of a potential to charge inflated rates.

---

Any price changes should therefore always have a transparent rationale.

Moreover, these people aren't always as rich or in possession of as much disposable income as you may think they are, or as they appear. Therefore, it's best not to make any assumptions about the levels of anyone's wealth.

As with any client, they might ask for a 'deal' or a special offer at the outset, so it's sensible to have some realistic options ready. Alternatively, you could offer them additional services that add value for the same price. As a 'one-off', you could split one treatment into two shorter sessions, which they might happily take, and you would thereby avoid discounting or reducing your core prices.

Some have so much money that sometimes you don't understand why they can be so picky about prices, or how, in contrast, less rich people are so easy and generous with their money. I recommend you just accept anyone's attitude towards money. Make sure they're all aware of and ready to pay your private fees, including any available offer or discount you have available for them. Over the years, however, and regardless of their status or financial situation, most of these clients have proved to be very generous, pay on time and are pleasant to treat and to communicate with. They are often very reliable and mostly aim to stay fit and active.

It is worth going the extra mile for every new client at the very start of each treatment, such as providing the best, most efficient sessions during the first consultation so they can save time while receiving more value than they expected. What many of my clients definitely seem to lack these days is time, not necessarily money; keep this in mind and act accordingly.

# Clients with Complex Conditions

Clients with complex conditions that you may find difficult to deal with can make you feel uncomfortable as a practitioner in one way or another. They drain some of your energy, bring up negative emotions, complain about your services inside and outside your practice, and to you personally, and often spend more of your time than they actually pay for. This includes you answering long emails and texts, hosting free drop-in sessions, dealing with their complaints, and them expecting you to change your schedule.

Such clients may delay payment on purpose, manipulate you emotionally, disrespect your skills and prices and make you angry, thoughtful or anxious during and after a session. They may also damage your reputation, intentionally or not, or might hurt you physically or emotionally.

These clients, hard work as they appear to be, are not necessarily bad and negative people; they may not harm you or your business on purpose, but they can do so without even noticing.

They may suffer from chronic and extremely limiting diseases such as ankylosing spondylitis, rheumatoid arthritis, fibromyalgia or myalgic encephalomyelitis, which cause them lots of pain, distress and disabilities, making their lives difficult and miserable. In some cases, the autonomic nervous system itself may be overloaded, impaired, or operating out of its optimal balance. That's a clinical feature often associate with emotional features, multiple and unclear physical symptoms or unorganised complaints.

---

## Therefore, beware of tagging someone or their entire clinical case too quickly for being or acting 'difficult' or for being overly complex.

---

As a private practitioner, I always aim to treat different people without any sort of discrimination. Yet I would rather complete treatment cycles in a relatively short period and a minimum number of sessions. Clients like these may have clinical and personal situations that you don't always have the right resources to deal with at your practice.

They will often need you on a more regular basis, with no clear, definite or measurable outcome of improvement or regression. Similarly, some unsuccessfully treated clients who can't be cured in a typical solo private practice, or whom you failed to help, may act or react in similar manners.

Sometimes, when clients with or without complex conditions act difficult, they will give you a hard time if they decide to delay payments, so you have to chase them, or they may be too demanding, complain often, cancel appointments or regularly fail to show up at all. They project the impression that you might lose them, and you may well find it uncomfortable to confront their behaviour and resolve the problem. They will often decide to just ignore you if you request payment or make a general inquiry about their progress—sometimes for some length of time, which you might find rather insulting. When you face difficulty dealing with someone of a seemingly higher profile than yours, always remember, though, that underneath any fancy suit there's a human being like everyone else– physically and emotionally– and so you should fear nothing about them or their position. Stand your ground in front of them politely and respectfully, if needed.

Therefore, at times some ordinary clients may be classified as 'difficult' or 'complicated' to deal with, and for all sorts of the right reasons.

If they ask you to invoice their insurance policy, it can make the money side of the situation somewhat easier, but you need to watch carefully and decide whether this is a client you want to treat.

It is fair to say that sometimes you'll reach a point where you need to stop treating particular clients–those you know are going to give you too hard a time. Sometimes it can be a false impression, but with more and more experience your gut feeling will start to guide you reliably.

This is not a pleasant decision to make or thing to do, especially when most of them aren't even aware of how they act, how they behave or how they make you feel. They might be very good people and well-paying clients, which makes it even harder.

However, your capacity to deliver your service the way you believe you should is more important than anything else.

It can become particularly stressful and challenging if you lose the will to serve clients for a few hours, days or even weeks, spending time apologising to them and compensating them, and then even struggle to sleep at night as a result of it all.

In the worst case, you may need to deal with serious complaints that lead to litigation, though this is very rare. Nonetheless, I discuss it later on.

Dealing with clients who suffer from complex conditions or with regular clients who aren't exactly your ideal match can be challenging but can also be very rewarding and enriching in different ways.

If you have a valid professional reason to stop serving any of your clients, and if you explain it to them honestly and help them find an alternative service provider, they may well appreciate your efforts and might even recommend future clients to you.

If something more serious or particularly awkward happens, or if such a client is unhappy about something, you need to do whatever possible to calm the situation down and make sure they're not going to cause you or your reputation any harm.

You can achieve this by offering the client an alternative solution such as a referral to further medical support or deeper investigation into their problem if relevant—or just some refund as a last resort. Beyond this, you need to make a quick and appropriate decision, based on the actual situation, about what action to take. Yet, from the very start, you should leave no room for the situation to escalate. Be aware of how the client feels and of when a situation has the potential to deteriorate.

To discharge people early yet effectively, one way is to explain that you can't help them anymore due to your limited knowledge and skills in the particular area of their complaints. You may just agree not to book another appointment for a long period of time, or you may simply refer them back to their GPs or to the right orthopaedic consultant—always with their consent.

Ideally, you shouldn't treat them again, and instead ensure they're happy to be referred to a colleague or to go back to their medical doctor or consultant for further examination.

There are many kinds of clients who you will find rather difficult to treat or deal with, and far more types of great clients who you'll build an excellent rapport with and find easy and pleasant to treat.

## Don't confuse difficult conditions with difficult personalities.

You can still get paid through helping wonderful people by diagnosing, advising, referring and relieving their symptoms, even if their overall condition doesn't fit directly with your MSKP/MT field of specialty.

You will gradually discover which types are good for you and which aren't. This is all about being able to help your clients and learning to enjoy helping everyone coming through your door.

# Dealing with Difficult Clients

The previous sections dealt with people who have complex conditions, which makes it potentially more difficult to treat them, and people who you'd find difficult to handle regardless of their physical request for help. I consider who these clients might be and what to expect from them.

Now I'd like to supply you with ideas about how to deal with the clients you don't wish to see anymore.

Among these clients are those who:

- Drain your mental and physical energy.
- Insult you on purpose.
- Harm your reputation.
- May have a 'crush' on you, and do not observe the physiotherapist–client relationship.
- Constantly take up far too much of your time and effort every session.
- You don't feel or think you can trust.
- You are sure you can't help.
- Don't pay on time once too often.
- Are friends or people whom you wish to become real friends with.
- You feel attracted to.

The best way to stop seeing clients without hurting their feelings is not necessarily to say how you feel when you treat them. Although it was mentioned previously, I wish to reiterate that most of them aren't even aware of how they behaved or if they've overreacted.

Some of them are well-paying clients who refer other good clients to you. For short-term clients, do your best to complete their treatment and discharge them. However, if the treatment is continuing, and you recognise features of a client type listed above, then simply review the situation. You can decide to continue, or you may say that you're struggling to make a difference and advise them to see someone else. Some of your colleagues will be delighted to take them on.

---

## Be honest. Make it clear you can't help your client's particular condition and that their current situation is outside your specialty.

---

Some new enquiries can be related to medico-legal cases. These are clinical or medical situations or injuries where a solicitor and an ongoing legal process are involved for the purpose of paying treatment expenses and/or other compensation.

Unless you specialise in such cases, obtain the client's consent and contact a practitioner who deals with such cases or conditions and refer them on. The administration and additional work are sometimes not worth it. Remember that you need to see clients who you can help quickly–ideally in a small number of sessions. The nature of the symptoms such clients often present you with is the 'whiplash' type, and they often present with chronic features. They won't be easy to diagnose, quick to fix or be ones with a clear clinical presentation. If something becomes a long-lasting episode, it may not be suitable for the type of practice you wish to build up for yourself. An exception would be existing clients whom you have seen and helped before and who now need your professional services under more complicated clinical circumstances such as complex fractures, or after orthopaedic surgery, where longer-term rehabilitation will be needed. It would be a perfectly fine and appropriate decision to help them out to the very best of your abilities.

Overall, you should simply disconnect yourself from such clients, the ones you find it emotionally or professionally difficult to engage with or help, but in the most professional and gentlest way possible. The approach is similar to quitting a job. Always do so professionally and remain on as good terms as possible.

If you wish to see a client in person–or ask them out, to create a natural friendship or for whatever other reason–it's often easiest to simply discharge that client. Start off by just telling them that for professional reasons you need to close their case and discharge them officially on your notes as well. Your client will probably agree to be discharged if there's the possibility of developing a more personal relationship.

# Avoiding Complaints and Dealing with Them

Client complaints, when not expressed aggressively or destructively, are always important; in fact, they may be giving you crucial information about how you can improve your services. However, clients' complaints can also ruin your reputation and business–or at least cause you lots of discomfort and stress. As a private physiotherapist, you may find that your clients, who have pain or an ongoing condition on the one hand, but who need to pay you on the other, may become emotionally unpredictable.

A small mistake–something you say, or any stressful situation the clients might be facing, whether linked or not to their physical problem–can lead to verbal or even physical aggression towards you.

Another contributing factor can be a delayed recovery. You may not have managed the problem effectively, perhaps due to the pathology itself, or because the client has not followed your advice.

# A problem that lasts longer than expected doesn't help any client –therapist relationship.

You'll need to identify problems accurately and share your findings with your client. Then always stay a step ahead of the situation.

For instance, if a paying client has come back to you for a third session and has reported no change at all to signs and symptoms, this should act as an alarm bell to you about their dissatisfaction. As an instant rule for you, start by re-examining their condition thoroughly, and you'll both often discover significant clinical changes such as the actual pain level and frequency, key muscle strength, mobility of joints and previously measured functional progress.

Never ignore complaints about the treatment progress becoming plateaued or making the situation worse, which might then turn into future complaints in person or, in the worst case, publicly.

This can happen even if you charge the right prices, have the right clinical skills and operate up to the expected clinical level, as I've explained throughout this book.

You can do a few things to prevent complaints and to deal effectively with those that do come in about your treatment's effectiveness and the value for money paid by the client:

## At the outset of any treatment...

- Present the signs and symptoms in writing or draw them at your initial consultation so that later you can easily compare, demonstrate or explain positive progress as well as relapses and regressions. Review and document the client's situation and progress thereafter and in detail during every treatment session.

## After the complaint: taking stock...

- Express concern that your client isn't recovering as expected.
- Repeat some of your examination procedures and explain what you're doing.
- Demonstrate some positive clinical progress that the client hasn't noticed.
- Repeat and demonstrate the unchanged parts of your treatment exactly as before.
- Give the client overall structural, functional, and social/contextual explanations about why parts of the treatment are unchanged.

## After the complaint: looking forward...

- Set specific and measured targets for your client for the next appointment.
- Identify any red flag (serious or warning pathology) or yellow flag (social or personal contributory factors) on account of which you would need to refer the client for further examination.
- If the situation escalates online or over the phone, then immediately offer a full review, re-examination or additional treatment at no charge to try to understand and help the situation.
- Ask them if there's anything else you can do for them or if they wish to get some of their money back and take it to try treatment elsewhere. They're most likely to agree to this offer and just move on at no additional harm to anyone.

If you follow these points, you will deal with the situation in the most effective way possible, and the client will trust you and pay your fees– even if you can't make them better. They may even recommend you to peers, knowing you left no stone unturned to help them out.

Another situation that can cause complaints is lateness, cancelling appointments at short notice, and making mistakes in your billing.

---

# Any obvious mistake you've made or an act of yours that causes even the slightest inconvenience to your patient must be followed up with an apology in writing, verbally, or face to face.

---

You might even offer compensation, such as a free treatment, or a full refund in more extreme situations–when the client has paid for the treatment privately. But though you may choose the right action, you shouldn't expect to continue as if nothing has happened.

In nearly all these situations, however, offer your sincere apologies and admit your fault if it will help to calm the situation down. You may want to just acknowledge any misunderstanding and discomfort caused to your client, and this will often be more than enough to settle an aggravated situation.

In extreme situations, such as when someone sends an email complaint, shouts at you or threatens you, it's wise to avoid the urge to react instantly and fight your own corner and to first listen to (or read the complaint) calmly and then get to the root of the issue. Explain your side of the story clearly and, if you don't wish to see them again, offer to refund the fee immediately because of their dissatisfaction with your service. Do so even if you feel they don't deserve it, as it should close their case officially. Although it's often helpful to admit your own fault, there will also be times when it's unwise to do so, for example, if the client seems particularly aggressive or, going by your previous experience, overly concerned with money. If in doubt, consult your professional body's solicitor immediately.

Keep any documentation of the conversation, and if you feel there's the slightest chance that a complaint may escalate into professional negligence, or a legal case – or if you sense a hint of them referring it to a sexual insult or assault–consult your professional organisation immediately too.

A common situation that may leave your client unsatisfied is when you take on a trainee or assistant to work with or observe you. Some clients may feel their privacy is being violated or that you are the only person who is entitled to treat them.

There is an earlier section in this book (Chapter 3) about trainees and assistants, but be aware that some patients may not want someone else, an additional male or female practitioner, to be present during their treatment, let alone treat them. It can be done properly, though, if agreed in advance and discounted when the trainee treats paying clients; if the patient also benefits from it in terms of having more detailed analysis; and if the service is more enhanced than in a normal session.

You might want to consider providing a targeted discount for integrating a trainee; your client might be delighted to receive a well-supervised treatment at a lower rate.

You could also include a clause in your initial consent form specifying that trainees and internal education are part of the regular operation of your practice.

Manual treatments require touching clients, and no matter how well trained you are, it is important to be prepared to deal with unpleasantness that may create discomfort or embarrassment for any of your clients. Make a special effort to avoid situations such as asking a client to get undressed in a cold room or forgetting to close the blinds of a window to protect your client's privacy.

If you mistakenly hurt someone physically, you must take action immediately. If at all possible, discuss the situation with your client, provide or arrange full medical care as needed, and reassure them that you are looking after them. Then contact your indemnity insurance provider for further instructions.

(Every healthcare practitioner is obliged to purchase insurance that provides such a service. It is often included in the membership fees of most healthcare professional, national chartered societies and regulating bodies.)

Once you've received their advice contact the client again.

You should not overcommunicate compensation, though you must certainly apologise for their inconvenience and reassure them that the case is being dealt with professionally.

You may give the client a refund for the entire treatment if they have already paid for it, though this depends on the situation and only applies if this repayment confirms the situation has been improved or even resolved between the two of you.

Promising to activate your insurance so you can provide the best compensation available may prevent further litigation against you, but you should do so only after getting approval from your professional body representative.

In nearly every case, you will be covered and insured, even in situations where you were at fault–or even negligent. Assuming that you did not act with criminal intent and you cannot be accused of a physical or sexual offence, any action a client may choose to take should not affect you dramatically. This is obviously apart from the clear loss of time and the inconvenience of dealing with it all.

---

## Always make sure you are paying the relevant professional bodies to cover your professional registration and indemnity insurance.

---

Finally, there are so many different professional scenarios that can spiral out of control and land you in serious problems. It is up to you to remain alert and professionally efficient so that you can detect potential flashpoints and react appropriately as they happen.

# Looking After Your Clients

This may sound trivial and basic, but looking after your clients is one of the most sensible and essential principles to adopt when running a private physiotherapy practice.

This is not to say that you should undervalue yourself or your services to please your clients. Don't extend sessions, give unwarranted discounts, or present your fees with an apologetic and humble tone–though I freely admit that from time to time I haven't taken my own advice.

To guide you on this subject more specifically, I list below a few do's (there are no don'ts) important points about serving your clients equally and appropriately:

- Be on time, especially on the first appointment. It is acceptable to be five or ten minutes late–as long as you acknowledge the delay, inform your client in advance, and clearly apologise.
- Reschedule appointments in advance or offer a refund for appointments you've failed to attend at the last moment.
- Be approachable during and between sessions.
- Identify the client's character and attitude and then act in a subtle way, using hints that would match their traits in a pleasant and genuine way. You can still be yourself, but understand who's in front of you and act in a way that would encourage them to be more open and feel more comfortable.
- Be clear about your fees and never adjust them without a clear explanation.
- Be accurate and informative during every session.
- Give good value, which also means providing a better understanding of the body's functions and its direct relation to your patient's problem.
- Diagnose treatable signs and symptoms, then attend to them immediately.

- Provide a detailed plan of how you're going to deal with each element of the problem.
- Show interest in your clients, listen to them, and remain communicative.
- Discuss their future schedule for additional bookings and follow-ups.

Most important of all is that your clients should be pleased with your services such that they're willing to pay your fees in return for high value for money. In this way, they will return and refer your services to their peers.

The ultimate value for money is reached by satisfying your client's initial expectations of what you discussed with them about the realistic goals you set together during the subjective part of the first consultation.

Satisfying those expectations is, in my view, the essential element of what 'looking after' your clients means.

# Attracting and Inspiring Clients

As a private practitioner, you need to first attract clients to your practice and then to positively inspire them as you deliver your services. This is not to say you should seduce them and take advantage of them in any way; that would lead to serious problems.

By 'attracting' and 'inspiring', I mean that people should a) be motivated to see you and leave your practice only when they feel better; b) be inspired to work harder on their bodies; and c) be motivated to become healthier and happier.

Your practice should be inspiring and should capture your clients' imagination, playing to the five senses. They should see, hear, smell and feel inspiration where possible. As for tasting, there are many options: offering a cup of good quality coffee or tea as they wait for their session or providing a healthy snack on the way out.

Alternatively, you can offer relevant educational material or a sample of pain-relieving rub or cream. This can be very helpful and show that you think, invest and care more during the first consulting session.

Sensory inspiration can also include simple things like agreeable aromas, soft, clean colours, professional decoration, attractive or inspiring pictures, pleasant music, and the feel of your own hands as needed.

You need to learn some principles of connecting with all kinds of people: simple actions that make people feel comfortable with you and like you enough to want to come back and see you regardless of the price you charge or how busy they are.

I want to add one caveat: never manipulate your clients emotionally in any way. If a client becomes attracted to you personally or romantically and the situation goes beyond the therapist–client relationship, you should acknowledge it and then–kindly and carefully– cease seeing this particular client professionally.

Any relationship between you and your clients must be one of friendly appreciation and trust: an integral part of the professional service you provide them with.

Your clients visit you with the aim of achieving a particular solution to their problem–not to get attention, find friendship, or seek a romantic relationship.

Yet professional relationships sometimes begin to enter the personal sphere. Should this start to happen, cease treatment, officially discharge the client and provide a referral to someone else. Only then should you explore a personal relationship.

It is all about your interaction, which should be based on a friendly, supportive and professional attitude. Without these you limit your chances of building up a successful private practice.

Applying this attitude to your work and to the people you serve will always attract and inspire more and more people in need of your skills and the services you can offer.

# 9 – AFTERWORDS

## Your Future

I n this book I describe a dream common to most physiotherapy students and graduate physiotherapists: opening a private practice and working for themselves, making a decent living and enjoying independence in their workplace. This is surely a worthwhile dream to pursue.

In reality, there's a long way to go before this dream can actually become a reality. I have failed a few times along the way, professionally and financially, before getting onto the right track and practising in the manner and in the environment of my choice as a private practitioner.

To achieve my dream, I had to leave my home country to study physiotherapy in the Netherlands. What's more, I had to learn Dutch from scratch so I could work there as a physiotherapist and treat the local population. Once I'd finished my studies and felt comfortable, I had to move again–this time to Glasgow in Scotland–and start all over again in English. (Looking back, English was certainly easier than Dutch.)

In Glasgow I immediately went back to university, enrolling on a part-time master's degree pathway in a system with which I was unfamiliar. After five years of working while studying part-time , I earned a postgraduate degree and a Master of Science (MSc) in Manual Therapy, which, as Musculoskeletal Physiotherapy, is a worldwide recognised specialty in this field.

While I was studying, I worked in a large clinic and then opened three different small practices, one after the other. They either failed or didn't work to my satisfaction. I kept starting up all over again, spending and losing lots of my own money along the way.

For my final attempt, I set up something far bigger and far more ambitious than I could handle. I had a viable business plan, and I employed another physiotherapist to help me build a brand-new clinic. Then, not long afterwards, we encountered serious cash-flow issues, partly due to my own limited managerial skills at the time.

I had to let my newly qualified physiotherapist employee go to recover financial losses, then start again, having virtually nothing apart from my recognised skills, reputation and a great client database of loyal clients to trade with.

Practising a profession I love while helping people every day made everything easier and worth all the setbacks to eventually succeed and realise my all-time dream.

You may wish to learn from my story, create your own pathway to success and avoid at least some of the pitfalls that I have recalled in this book. Take my advice if you like and remember that you can fulfil similar dreams and do even better to get there even sooner—if you are dedicated and focused.

What you'll get at the end is a sense of professional achievement and job satisfaction while enjoying a level of financial and job security that very few people, particularly physiotherapists, ever get in their working life.

It is up to you to take the first step towards professional freedom. Go back to the previous chapters, take some notes and start up your future career as a private physiotherapist.

Remember that this book is not about achieving financial freedom, and it is not a prescription for a happy millionaire lifestyle. You will be disappointed if you expected to find a quick fix in this regard.

---

# You'll need to work hard to earn your professional freedom first before getting any chance for financial freedom.

---

Then you will need to go on working hard to keep yourself there and work on making the money and lifestyle that you want for yourself and your family.

However, if you decide to take the next step and build up a larger business to achieve full financial freedom, then once you've finished this book you'll be in a far better position professionally–and soon financially–to do so.

Alternatively, you could enjoy an attractive and rewarding professional and financial life if you decide to keep working by yourself alone in your own practice. I still love it and it opens massive new opportunities on a regular basis.

During my journey, I've met physiotherapists from around the world who kept their business on a small scale, and I was very surprised at the quality of the personal and family life they had developed alongside this.

## We are in the era when money can be made in more informative ways and not only through treating clients back-to-back.

Our accumulated knowledge, skills and often our inspirational behaviour can be fairly easily monetised to serve many more people than the ones we are treating in person. Just take this book that you're reading right now as a simple example of this.

# The Future of Private Physiotherapy

We are physiotherapists who practise an evidence-based profession, which means decisions and actions are based on the best available, current, valid and relevant research. A profession that belongs to a nationally recognised healthcare system along with other allied health professions. Yet we shouldn't forget that we have no monopoly on treating the human body, especially when it comes to treating movement disorders and sports injuries.

We should keep our eyes, ears and minds open to other healthcare providers with approaches different from our own. We should meet, listen, and learn from each other and maintain an overall respect for other professionals.

# Some professions deal with similar dysfunctions and have truly great methods that we can learn from.

Osteopaths, chiropractors, sports therapists, kinesiologists, alternative therapists, masseurs–and even bodyworkers who don't possess any recognised or academic qualifications at all– may sometimes astonish you with their skills and abilities to improve and remove symptoms.

It is sometimes hard for us to recognise other practitioners because they may not always value us in the same way.

Take, for example, an average chiropractor who works in a fancy-looking suit, styles himself or herself 'X–doctor of chiropractic' and treats clients by manipulating their spine for an entire session that lasts no longer than a few minutes. How much more efficient could any collaboration be?

These professionals may not feel there's much point in forming a community of practice with an average physiotherapist who dresses up in branded sports clothes and treats clients mostly by exercising muscles and is often 'scared' to manipulate spinal joints, for sessions that may last up to an hour each.

It can also happen the other way around, when a physiotherapist is obliged to perform comprehensive examinations followed by evidence-based treatment. While such treatment involves carefully selected muscular training and manipulative methods based on a detailed clinical process, what does he or she have in common with chiropractor Doctor X? Someone who just adopts the title 'Doctor' having never graduated from medical school and often possessing no more than four years of non-academic studies may well not be a suitable candidate for potential collaboration.

Despite all this, we should always remember that we are all students throughout our life-long career, and we can always learn from others. Go out and meet professionals you might consider competitors and learn from them.

Ignore titles, recognitions or previous concepts you or your peers may have about other practitioners. Feel comfortable communicating with them all. Approach your career as a learning curve.

After studying some of the original sources of our profession and other allied health and alternative healthcare professions from the past, I truly believe that one day we can all practise a selection–or mix–of the same methods, and perhaps develop similar educational and professional programmes. Physiotherapists, chiropractors and osteopaths not only share some similar background history but also often start to explore and even start to adopt each other's knowledge and practical or clinical skills.

I admit that some of the best techniques and then entire professional approaches I have seen, studied or experienced were not necessarily accepted and practised by Western physiotherapists, but they were based, nonetheless, on very similar professional backgrounds.

However, in my experience, MSKP/MT includes knowledge, skills, clinical reasoning process and an evidence base to achieve great results. We also live in a field of rapidly developing technology which, as discussed earlier, should not be ignored by practitioners of any healthcare profession.

We can help our clients to get there safely, in a short time, and with long-lasting results.

Add to it genuine client care and a personal approach to make physiotherapy an ultimate platform to deliver excellent services in private practice.

Keep learning, develop yourself, grow your own practice and provide a great service to help as many people as you can.

Enjoy your practice,
Gal.

# THE POST COVID-19 PRIVATE PRACTICE

T he content of this book refers to private practice work in general; it was written over a long professional period of years, mostly prior to the pandemic, so it doesn't take into account COVID-19, nor can it predict global circumstances in the future. However, some sections in it have been slightly modified with relevant references to this rather long-lasting pandemic.

As such, I don't discuss social distancing, hands-on limitations in treatment or the many other restrictions and rules that had to be adopted in a private practice for a while. Everyone needs to take responsibility for following national and professional guidelines.

This book delivers an overall approach to practising physiotherapy privately, provided you're fully qualified, registered and allowed to do so. COVID-19 and healthcare regulations in general differ according to countries, regions and professions, and you need to be clear about whether the licences, education and equipment you need might have to be adapted to protect yourself and your clients. It is up to you to stay safe, well educated, legally registered, and up to date at all times.

However, the core knowledge in this book is largely applicable, even if it must be somewhat modified to account for the current situation, to deliver full value to your clients. Personal attitude, a professional approach, thorough clinical reasoning and safety during your sessions should still be prioritised and considered in your practice alongside the COVID-19 or any other future global health change.

The ways to build up, market and look after your practice and clients need only be updated according to current circumstances that you and your clients are facing.

Beyond the difficulties and overall inconvenience that COVID-19 has imposed on us all, it also held out great new opportunities for us to reinvent our professional and clinical excellence.

Reducing or eliminating the physical contact upon which your advanced knowledge and attitude in your practice is based can inspire new solutions to physical problems that your clients can't easily find elsewhere.

The world has changed and continues to evolve, but your clients or future clients are still there; they still expect good value despite any understandable limitations.

Physical problems can be improved and resolved, and pain can be relieved, with or without contacting patients physically and using your hands. As most COVID-19 restrictions gradually reduced, some of the treatment technologies discussed earlier on match the pandemic's general requirement of social distancing too, which is an added benefit. It's mainly about understanding the mechanism of pain and the background to any physical problem that opens the pathway to first explaining it clearly and then to resolving it.

Your ability to communicate effectively, build rapport and use clinical reasoning are already the most valuable building blocks you should use in private practice–before, during and post COVID-19.

Get a good understanding and mastery of these valuable elements, then go ahead to start practising it all–safely and effectively!

Stay well, active and safe–Gal.

www.ingramcontent.com/pod-product-compliance
Lightning Source LLC
Chambersburg PA
CBHW071552200326

41519CB00021BB/6720